For Sally and Michael

For Churchill Livingstone

Publisher: Lucy Gardner
Copy Editor: Holly Gothard
Production Controller: Mark Sanderson
Design: Design Resources Unit
Sales Promotion Executive: Kathy Crawford

100 Paediatric Picture Tests

A. P. Winrow
BSc (Hons) MB BS MRCP (UK)
Senior Registrar in Paediatrics, St Mary's Hospital, London

M. Gatzoulis
MD DCH
Fellow of the Greek Paediatric Association
Fellow in Paediatric Cardiology, Royal National Brompton Hospital, London

G. Supramaniam
MSc MB BS MRCP (UK)
Consultant Paediatrician, Watford General Hospital;
Honorary Consultant Paediatrician, St Mary's Hospital, London

CHURCHILL LIVINGSTONE
EDINBURGH LONDON MADRID MELBOURNE NEW YORK AND TOKYO 1994

CHURCHILL LIVINGSTONE
Medical Division of Longman Group UK Limited

Distributed in the United States of America by Churchill
Livingstone Inc., 650 Avenue of the Americas, New York,
N.Y. 10011, and by associated companies, branches and
representatives throughout the world.

First published 1994
  Reprinted 1994

ISBN 0-443-04942-4

British Library Cataloguing in Publication Data
A catalogue record for this book is available from the
British Library.

Library of Congress Cataloging in Publication Data
A catalog record for this book is available from the
Library of Congress.

The
publisher's
policy is to use
**paper manufactured
from sustainable forests**

Printed in Hong Kong
LYP/02

CONTENTS

Preface   vii

Questions and Answers 1–100   1–200

Index to Questions   201

Preface

The MRCP examination remains a significant and anxiety-provoking hurdle in the career of an aspiring clinician. The visual material section requires wide clinical experience. While it is not a substitute for such experience, this book is designed to supplement it and to serve as an adjunct to the candidate's revision programme.

The variety of cases, experienced by the authors, which appear in this book represent problems common to the MRCP and daily clinical practice. Although the spectrum of cases is extensive, it is not exhaustive, and we apologize for any omissions which have necessarily occurred. Most of the cases are accompanied by questions which examine the reader's knowledge of diagnosis and aspects of management. The majority are followed by short notes summarizing relevant important facts and supported by references to key reviews or recent original articles.

While some answers list differential diagnoses, there has been no attempt to score such answers, as this might mislead candidates into attempting to predict the examiners' marking schemes.

Although this book is aimed primarily at those undertaking the MRCP paediatric examination, we hope that it will also be of benefit to those studying for the Diploma in Child Health. Furthermore, the cases may be utilized as discussion material for problem-orientated tutorials in teaching programmes for medical students.

Should readers encounter any mistakes in the book, we would welcome comments and advice aimed at correcting them. We wish those labouring under the stress of examinations great success.

London, 1994

A.P.W.
M.G.
G.S.

Question 1

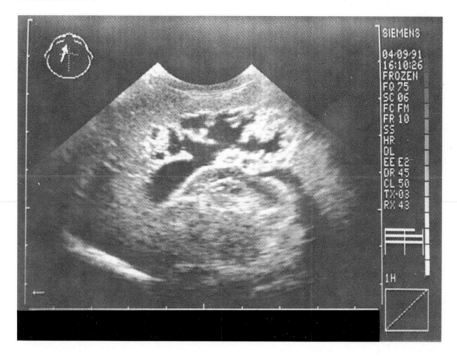

This is a cranial ultrasound scan of a 28 week gestation infant performed at 5 weeks of age.

a) What is the diagnosis?
b) What is the likely prognosis of such an ultrasound appearance?
c) This appearance was not detected on an earlier cranial scan performed on the second day of life. Why?

Answer to Question 1

a) Periventricular leucomalacia (PVL).
b) Guarded prognosis. Cerebral palsy may develop.
c) PVL results from progressive cavitation of early echodense lesions. Early scans may demonstrate signs of the causative insult but may be normal. PVL is rarely detected before 14 days of life by routine ultrasonography.

- PVL is a result of tissue necrosis following ischaemia or infarction.
- PVL is usually multicystic and these may coalesce.
- Changes in cerebral blood flow and perfusion have been implicated as aetiological factors. Hypovolaemia, asphyxia and pneumo-thoraces are some of the factors combining with poor cerebral perfusion autoregulation causing this problem.
- Occipitoparietal or bilateral PVL carries a worse prognosis.
- PVL may result in cerebral palsy, microcephaly, audiovisual and intellectual deficits. Long term follow-up is mandatory, preferably based within a multidisciplinary child development centre.
- Porencephaly is usually unicystic and is often in direct communication with the ventricular system. Prognosis may be better.

Levene M 1990 Cerebral ultrasound and neurological impairment: telling the future. Arch. Dis. Child. 65:469–471

Question 2

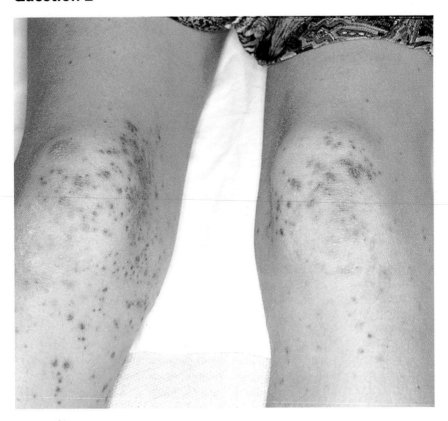

This skin rash was noted when an 11-year-old girl was admitted with generalized acute abdominal pain.

a) What is the diagnosis?
b) Give two possible causes for her abdominal pain.
c) List four potential complications of this condition.

Answer to Question 2

a) Henoch–Schönlein purpura (HSP)
b) Gut wall oedema and haemorrhage
   Acute intussusception
   Unrelated GI pathology
   Poorly localized hip pain
c) Arthropathy
   Renal disease: nephritis, nephrotic syndrome, renal failure
   CNS disease: seizures, paresis, rarely coma
   Testicular torsion
   Peripheral desquamation

- Vasculitic condition often preceded by an upper respiratory tract infection.
- Most common non-thrombocytopenic purpura.
- Probably IgA Type III immune complex reaction.
- Serum IgA and complement levels may be elevated.
- Rheumatoid factor and antinuclear factor negative.
- Purpura may be preceded by urticaria. Lower limb extensor surfaces are most commonly affected.
- Arthritis/arthralgia is usually transient and non-migratory.
- Renal involvement in 40–60%; renal failure ensues in 1%.
- Gross proteinuria is a poor prognostic indicator although moderate proteinuria and haematuria may persist for months.
- Treatment is symptomatic although steroids may ameliorate the abdominal pain.
- Schönlein described the triad of arthropathy, rash and GI manifestations. Henoch associated the rash, arthropathy and nephritis.

Graham-Pole J 1988 Henoch Schönlein purpura. In: Clayden G S, Hawkins R L (eds) Treatment and prognosis. Heinemann, London

Question 3

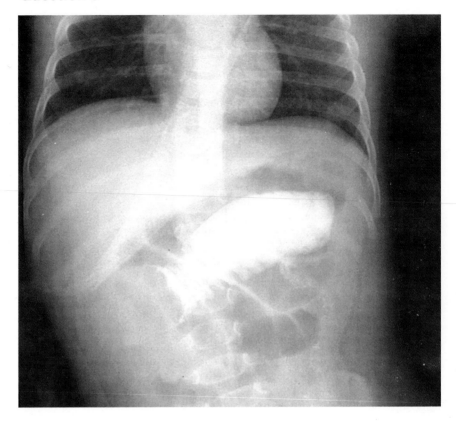

a) Name this radiological procedure.
b) What is the diagnosis?
c) Give two contra-indications to performing this procedure.

Answer to Question 3

a) Barium enema.
b) Acute intussusception.
c) Absolute contra-indications are evidence of perforation and peritonitis. Prolonged history (>24–48 hours) with evidence of GI bleeding
  is a relative contra-indication.

- Incidence 1–2/1000 live births.
- Classical age distribution is 4 to 18 months; preterm infants and
  older children may be affected.
- Aetiology: postviral or idiopathic. Polyps, Meckel diverticulum and
  lymphoma may occur in the older child.
- Typical history of paroxysmal screaming, episodic pallor, vomiting,
  pulling up of knees and the passage of redcurrant jelly stools may be
  absent. The latter is a late sign.
- Painless intussusception occurs in 13–20% of cases.
- Plain radiography may show fluid levels, small bowel dilatation and
  a paucity of gas shadows in the right iliac fossa.
- Ultrasound demonstrates the 'swiss roll' sign.
- Barium enema may illustrate the 'stack of coins' sign.
- Peritonitis, perforation, recurrence (4–10%) or failure of hydrostatic
  reduction (25%) are indications for surgery.
- Intussusception occurs in Henoch–Schönlein purpura.
- Chronic intussusception is a rare cause of failure to thrive.

Paes R A , Hyde I, Griffiths D M 1988 The management of intussusception. Br. J. Radiol. 61:187–189
Stringer M D, Pledger G, Drake D P 1992 Childhood deaths from
intussusception in England and Wales 1984–89. Br. Med. J.
304:737–739

Question 4

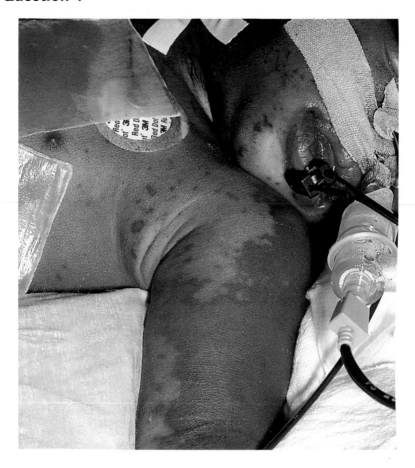

This 2-year-old girl collapsed at home and subsequently developed this rash.

a) Name this rash.
b) What is the most likely cause for this child's collapse?
c) What is the prognosis?

Answer to Question 4

a) Purpura fulminans.
b) Meningococcal septicaemia.
c) Poor prognosis. Regular assessment using the Glasgow Meningococcal Septicaemia Score (GMSS) aids management and helps to predict prognosis.

- The rash of meningococcaemia may vary from macular to classic purpura; the latter may coalesce and become haemorrhagic. Subsequent sloughing leaves ulcers.
- Mortality approximates to 20–40%.
- The major processes involved in meningococcal septicaemia are: increased vascular permeability leading to hypovolaemia; either vascular bed dilatation or vasoconstriction differing in various organs; intravascular thrombosis associated with clotting factor and platelet activation and consumption exacerbating tissue hypoxia and ischaemia.
- Admission to intensive care facilities when the GMSS >8.
- Activation of cytokines (e.g. elevated TNF, reduced prostacyclin) results in clinical deterioration despite antibacterial and supportive care.
- Positive blood cultures in <50%.
- Latex particle agglutination test is positive in 35–45%.
- Large volumes of colloids, inotropes and often ventilatory support are needed to maximize tissue perfusion and oxygenation.
- Prostacyclin may aid perfusion, oxygenation, fibrinolysis and inhibition of platelet activation. Antilipopolysaccharide endotoxin monoclonal antibodies may be beneficial.

Heyderman R S, Klein N J, Shennan G I, Levin M 1991 Deficiency of prostacyclin production in meningococcal shock. Arch. Dis. Child. 66:1296–1299
Sinclair J F, Skeoch C H, Hallworth D 1987 Prognosis of meningococcal septicaemia. Lancet ii:38

Question 5

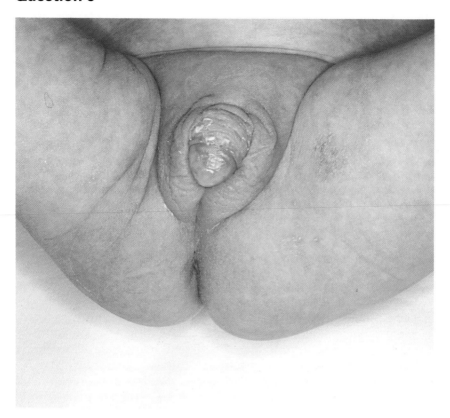

The above appearance was noted on the initial neonatal examination

a) What is the most likely diagnosis?
b) List four useful investigations to confirm the diagnosis.
c) Briefly outline your long term management of this child.

Answer to Question 5

a) Congenital adrenal hyperplasia.
b) Plasma 17 hydroxyprogesterone
Plasma 11 deoxycortisol
Karyotype
Plasma ACTH and plasma renin activity
Plasma testosterone and androstenedione
Pelvic ultrasonography
Urinary steroid assays.
c) Gluco- and mineralocorticoid replacement, often with salt supple-
mentation during infancy, aiming to maintain normal growth.
Monitoring of growth, bone age, blood pressure and biochemistry.
Reconstructive surgery. Psychological support.

- Most common enzyme abnormality is 21 hydroxylase deficiency.
- Complex autosomal recessive; chromosome 6p–two genes, A and
  B. The former is a pseudogene and the B gene is active. B gene
  deletion accounts for 25% of cases.
- Two thirds of sufferers are salt losers. The earliest indication is a
  rising potassium level at a median of 4 days.
- Initial replacement with glucocorticoids and salt supplements is
  modified by the introduction of mineralocorticoid. 17 hydroxyprogesterone (elevated) is a mineralocorticoid antagonist.
- Anthropometric assessment provides good results in terms of
  growth. These may be supplemented by measurement of biochemical indices but interpretation is complex due to diurnal
  changes.
- Bone age exceeding chronological age suggests undertreatment
  and vice versa.
- Plasma renin activity is a sensitive indicator of salt balance.
- Late onset disease may present with precocious puberty. Sub-
  fertility and delayed menarche may be due to associated polycystic
  ovaries.
- Antenatal diagnosis is available. Early use of dexamethasone in
  pregnancy may reduce fetal virilization.

Brook C G D 1990 The management of classical congenital adrenal
hyperplasia due to 21 hydroxylase deficiency. Clin. Endocrinol.
33:559–567

Question 6

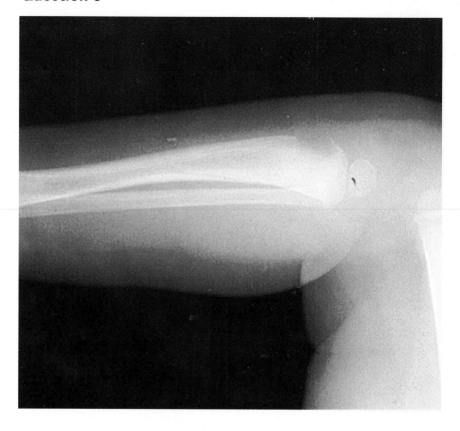

This is an X-ray of a neonate.

a) What is the diagnosis?
b) List four possible presentations of your diagnosis in a neonate.
c) What long term problem may be encountered?

Answer to Question 6

a) Tibial osteomyelitis.
b) Septicaemia
   Apnoea
   Limb pseudoparalysis
   Limb swelling
   Jaundice
   Non-specific problems, e.g. poor feeding, irritability.
c) Epiphyseal plate damage leading to deformity and discrepant limb growth.

- Term babies often present with pseudoparalysis and little systemic disturbance.
- Preterm infants may have multifocal disease; septicaemia is common. Pronounced leucocytosis is often present.
- Radiological changes occur early, particularly in the preterm infant when they may be present at diagnosis. Radiological resolution is usually complete.
- Radionuclide bone scans may be falsely negative.
- Causative organisms in the neonate: staphylococci, enterococci and streptococci.
- Septic arthritis occurs due to transphyseal spread.
- Fusidic acid is often added to the flucloxacillin/gentamicin antibiotic cover to reduce the emergence of resistant organisms. Supportive and surgical therapy may be required.

Williamson J B, Galasko C S B, Robinson M J 1990 Outcome of acute osteomyelitis in preterm infants. Arch. Dis. Child. 65:1060–1062

Question 7

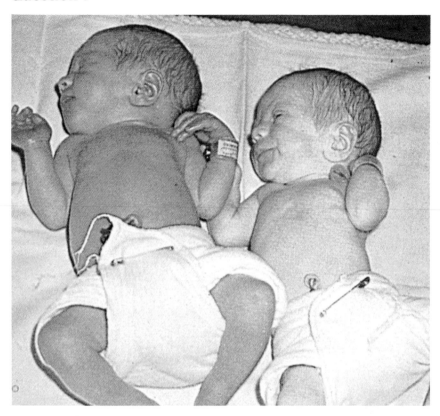

These twins were born at a gestation of 37 weeks.

a) Explain the different appearance of these babies.
b) What is the most important initial investigation?
c) List three potential complications of this phenomenon.

Answer to Question 7

a) Twin–twin transfusion
b) Spun haematocrit
c) Polycythaemic infant: hyperbilirubinaemia
                                    hypoglycaemia
                                    hypocalcaemia
                                    hyperviscosity syndrome
                                    acidosis
                                    thrombocytopenia
                                    cardiac failure

    Anaemic infant: cardiac failure
                                    hypo-albuminaemia
                                    poor growth

- Occurs in monozygous twins with shared placenta.
- Incidence 7% of twins.
- Chronic transfusion may cause stillbirth or birth weight discrepancy of 20%.
- Blood viscosity increases exponentially when the haematocrit is >65%.
- Hyperviscosity syndrome includes: respiratory distress
                                    jitteriness and seizures
                                    necrotizing enterocolitis
                                    renal vein thrombosis
                                    cerebral thrombosis.
- Plasma dilutional exchange transfusion is indicated if the venous haematocrit >65% or if the child is symptomatic. Capillary haematocrits exceed venous or arterial measurements.
- Paradoxical bone mineralization has been reported; osteopenia in the polycythaemic infant and osteosclerosis in the other.

Bishop N J, King F J, Ward P et al 1990 Paradoxical bone mineralisation in the twin to twin transfusion syndrome. Arch. Dis. Child. 65:705–706

Question 8

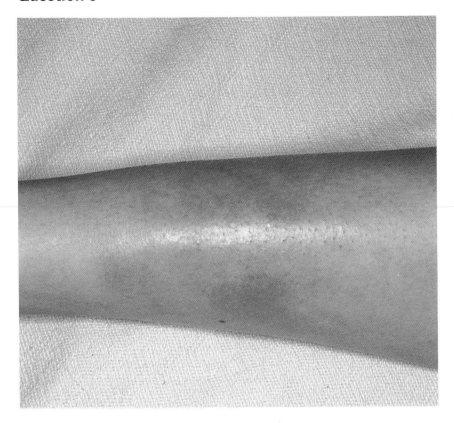

This teenage girl has acutely painful legs. She has recently suffered a mild cold. Her only medication is mefenamic acid and the oral contraceptive pill, both prescribed for her troublesome menorrhagia.

a) What is the diagnosis?
b) List six causes.
c) What is the treatment?

Answer to Question 8

a) Erythema nodosum (EN)
b) Infection: streptococcal
                  mycoplasmal
                  mycobacterial
                  enteric–salmonella, yersinia, etc.
                  parasites
                  viral–EBV, varicella, herpes
   Drugs: sulphonamides, contraceptive pill
   Inflammatory bowel disease
   Sarcoidosis
   SLE
c) Reassurance and analgesia. Severe and recurrent disease may be treated with both steroids and indomethacin.

- EN is rare below 6 years of age.
- Female preponderance.
- Lesions are red, indurated, shiny, painful and symmetrical.
- Lesions fade as bruises but residual hyperpigmentation may persist.
- Pathology: immune complex mediated reactions in the sub-cutaneous tissues around large vessels producing nodules and plaques, predominantly over the tibial aspects.
- Relapsing cases may have IgG2 subclass deficiency.
- There have been notable sufferers–Mozart reputedly suffered from EN when 6 years old.

Question 9

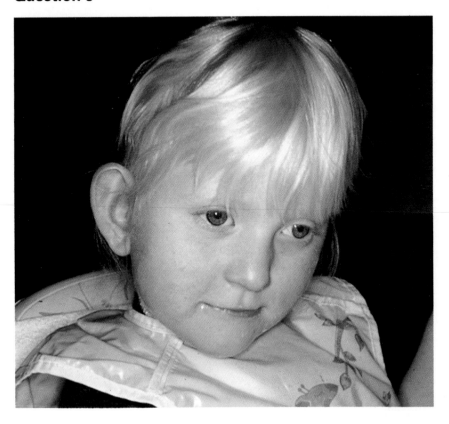

The above child has global developmental delay and is prone to unprovoked paroxysmal laughter.

a) What is the most likely diagnosis?
b) List three other associated features.
c) How is this condition inherited?

Answer to Question 9

a) Angelman syndrome ('happy puppet')
b) Seizures, jerky ataxia, brachycephaly, wide mouth and jaw prominence
c) Genomic imprinting with uniparental disomy.

- Described by Angelman in 1965.
- No pathognomic features but many have blond hair and blue eyes.
- 90% have seizures. The EEG is abnormal with a slow wave cycle of 4–6 per second.
- 70% have severe retardation, language deficits and microcephaly.
- CT brain scans may be normal or show mild cerebral atrophy.
- Gait is broad based.
- Genetic abnormality: 15q 11–13 (maternal deletion).
- Uniparental disomy occurs when both alleles are inherited from one parent. This may account for the differences between Angelman syndrome and Prader–Willi syndrome, both of which result from similar deletions but of chromosomes inherited from the other parent.

Clayton–Smith J 1992 Angelman's syndrome. Arch. Dis. Child. 67:889–891
Hall J G 1990 Genomic imprinting. Arch. Dis. Child. 65:1013–1016
Robb S A, Pohl K R E, Baraitser M et al 1989 The 'happy puppet' syndrome of Angelman: review of the clinical features. Arch. Dis. Child. 64:83–86

Question 10

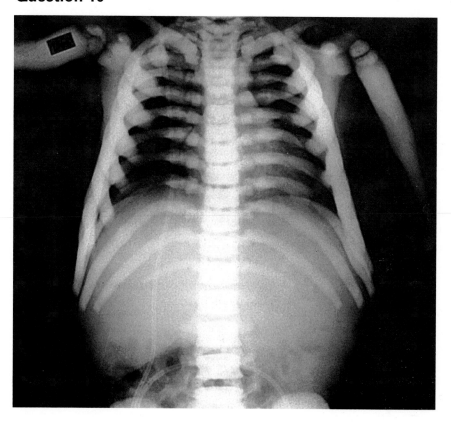

An Asian child is referred with hepatosplenomegaly. Moderate anaemia, thrombocytopenia, metamyelocytes and normoblasts were noted on blood film and marrow aspiration analysis. This is her chest radiograph.

a) What is the diagnosis?
b) What diagnostic clue was noted during the marrow aspiration?
c) List three complications of your diagnosis.

Answer to Question 10

a) Osteopetrosis (marble bone or Albers–Schönberg disease)
b) 'Dry-tap' or difficult marrow aspiration
c) Blindness, hearing deficits, hydrocephalus, cranial nerve palsies, bone fractures, marrow failure and recurrent sepsis

- Inheritance: severe (autosomal recessive); benign (dominant).
- Failure of osteoclast resorption with persistence of primary calcified cartilaginous matrix and defective bone remodelling resulting in osteosclerosis.
- Bony foramina fail to develop thus causing nerve palsies and hydrocephalus.
- Spinal X-rays show a 'rugby jersey' pattern and long bones demonstrate 'clubbed' metaphyses.
- Hepatosplenomegaly, jaundice and failure to thrive occur.
- Treatment is largely supportive; steroids are not consistently of benefit. Bone marrow transplantation is potentially curative since the graft supplies new stem cell derived osteoclasts. There is a high incidence of graft rejection and results may be limited by previous neurological problems.

Watson A C H 1992 Disorders of bone. In: Cambell AGM, McIntosh N (eds) Forfar and Arneil's textbook of paediatrics, 4th edn. Churchill Livingstone, Edinburgh

Question 11

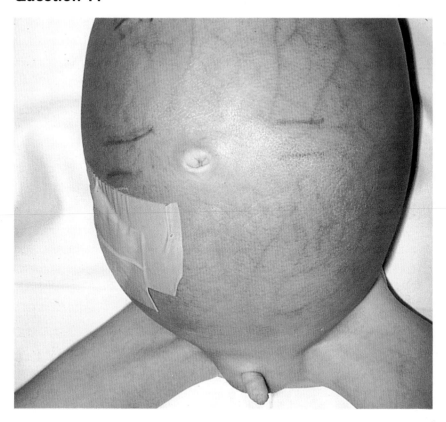

a) List three abnormal physical signs apparent in this slide.
b) What diagnostic procedure has been performed in the right iliac fossa?
c) What is the possible relationship between this picture and this infant's hydrocephalus?

Answer to Question 11

a) Abdominal distension due to ascites
   Prominent dilated anterior abdominal wall vessels
   Umbilical eversion
   Right subchondral scar following ventriculoperitoneal shunt
   insertion
b) Diagnostic paracentesis
c) Sclerosing peritonitis

- Sclerosing peritonitis is a rare complication of CSF drainage into the peritoneal cavity via a shunt.
- Ascitic fluid analysis may be misleading and is a mixture of CSF and exudate. It is usually sterile.
- Peritoneal biopsy shows evidence of chronic inflammation.
- Other causes of ascites must be excluded, particularly fungal infections and mycobacterial infections.
- Radionuclide studies demonstrate shunt patency although peritoneal absorptive capacity may be diminished.
- Conversion of shunt to a ventriculo-atrial type has been advocated.

Question 12

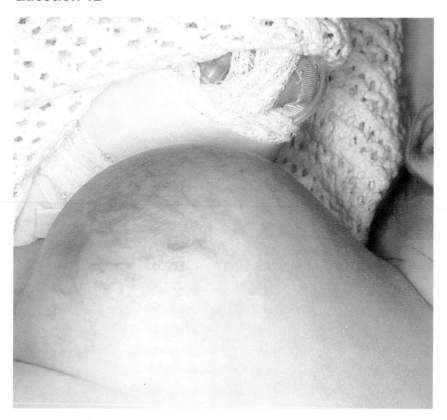

The abnormality pictured above has been present since birth.

a) What is the diagnosis?
b) What investigation will confirm your diagnosis?
c) Give two potential complications.

Answer to Question 12

a) Thoracic lymphangioma
b) Ultrasound ('bunch of grapes' picture)
c) Sepsis and haemorrhage

- Developmental abnormality of lymphatic origin.
- Endothelial cell lining.
- Most common site affected is the neck (cystic hygroma).
  Others include: lip, tongue, axilla and groin.
- Complications depend upon the location: obstructed labour, tracheal compression, difficulty in mastication and deglutition.
- Surgery is hazardous due to the risk of haemorrhage or the involvement of deeper structures. Several tissue planes may be involved.

Watson A C H 1992 Surgical paediatrics. In: Campbell A G M, McIntosh N (eds) Forfar and Arneil's textbook of paediatrics, 4th edn. Churchill Livingstone, Edinburgh

Question 13

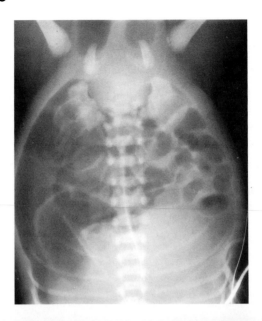

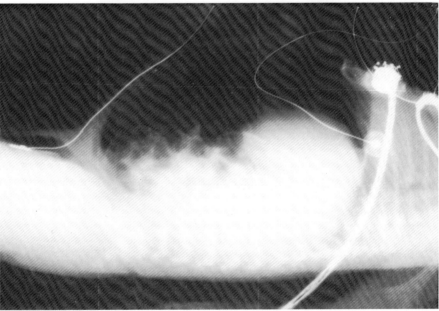

A severely asphyxiated preterm infant deteriorated with abdominal distension and acidosis whilst receiving mechanical ventilation. These abdominal X-rays were obtained.

a) List three abnormal radiological features.
b) What is the most likely diagnosis?
c) Why was a rectal biopsy performed in the convalescent period?

Answer to Question 13

a) Free intraperitoneal gas
   Thickened oedematous loops of bowel
   Intrascrotal gas (via a patent processus vaginalis)
b) Necrotizing enterocolitis (NEC)
c) Exclusion of Hirschsprung disease which may present with acute
   enterocolitis (15%)

- NEC may affect up to 35% of preterm infants. It can occur in term
  infants.
- Multifactorial aetiology: asphyxia, shock, sepsis and early, particu-
  larly formula, feeds.
- Mortality 40%; surgery in 20% and late GI strictures in 10%.
- Antenatal absent or reversed end diastolic flow velocities on
  Doppler studies of umbilical arteries may predict those at risk of
  NEC.
- NEC is associated with patent ductus arteriosus and indomethacin
  therapy. This may be due to indomethacin administration causing
  exacerbation of splanchnic hypoperfusion, due to the ductus,
  resulting in NEC.
- X-ray abnormalities include: fixed dilated oedematous loops of
  bowel, pneumatosis intestinalis, perforation and intrabiliary gas.
- Clostridial species have been implicated in 20% of cases.
- Management entails supportive therapy, antibiotics and cessation
  of feeds with the introduction of parenteral nutrition.

Coombs R C, Morgan M, Durbin G et al 1990, Gut blood flow velocities
in the newborn: effects of patent ductus arteriosus and parenteral
indomethacin. Arch. Dis. Child. 65:1067–1071

Question 14

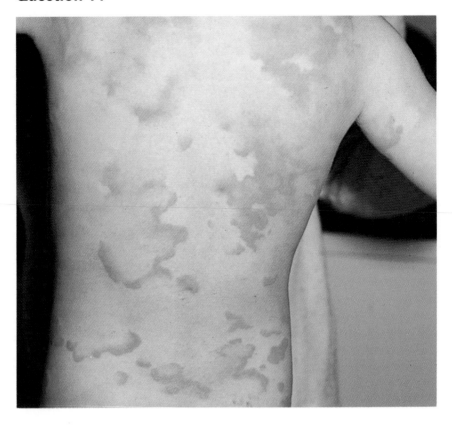

a) What is the diagnosis?
b) In which multisystem disorder may this physical sign occur?

Answer to Question 14

a) Erythema marginatum
b) Acute rheumatic fever

- Erythema marginatum comprises erythematous rings with pale centres of normal skin. These frequently coalesce and may vary in conformation during the day.
- It only occasionally appears in acute rheumatic fever and is then considered to constitute a major criterion.
- Other major criteria include: polyarthritis
  carditis
  subcutaneous nodules
  rheumatic chorea.

Question 15

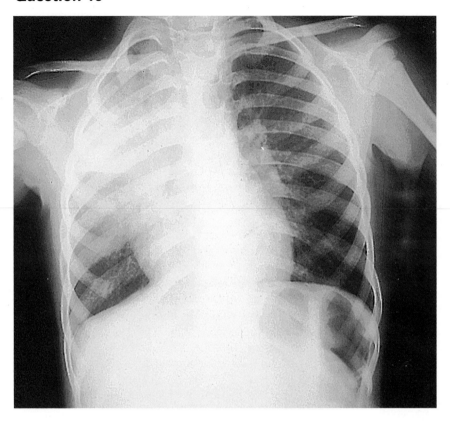

A 6-year-old girl with homozygous sickle cell disease presented with fever and respiratory failure. This is her chest radiograph.

a) Give two possible diagnoses.
b) List three measures designed to prevent these diagnoses.

Answer to Question 15

a) Right upper lobe pneumonia
Sickle chest syndrome
b) Penicillin prophylaxis
Antipneumococcal vaccination
High transfusion policy to maintain low HbSS concentrations

- Sickle chest syndrome may present with acute breathlessness and pain. It may mimic pneumonia on the chest X-ray.
- Sickle chest syndrome comprises changes of sequestration, infarction and subsequent consolidation.
- Encapsulated organisms, e.g. pneumococcus and haemophilus, are common and the risk of sepsis is 600 times that of the unaffected population.
- Defective immunocompetence occurs due to defective opsonization and hyposplenism.
- Antipneumococcal vaccination is recommended for those over 2 years of age and penicillin prophylaxis for those over 3 months.
- Acute exchange transfusion is required during sickle chest and neurological crises to reduce HbSS levels, reduce secondary sickling and aid oxygenation.
- Following such crises, high transfusion policies may have to be continued indefinitely to avoid recurrence.

Evans J P M 1989 Practical management of sickle cell disease. Arch. Dis. Child. 64:1748–1751
Haupt H M, Moore G W, Bauer T W et al 1982 The lung in sickle cell disease. Chest 81:332–337

Question 16

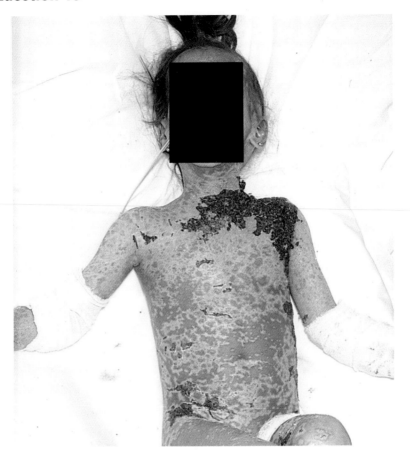

This sick child exhibits a severe dermatological condition.

a) What is the diagnosis?
b) Give three potential complications.
c) Briefly outline your management.

Answer to Question 16

a) Eczema herpeticum
b) Dissemination of herpes simplex
Encephalitis
Secondary bacterial infection
c) Parenteral and topical acyclovir
Broad spectrum, including antistaphylococcal, antibiotics

- Lesions may become haemorrhagic.
- Ocular complications may occur.
- Secondary sepsis is common.

Question 17

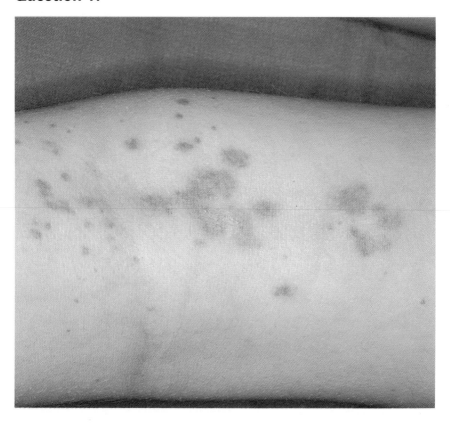

The above rash was noted in a child with neck stiffness and fever. The child subsequently developed petechiae.

a) What is the most likely diagnosis?
b) How does the prognosis vary in comparison with the usual presentation of this condition?

Answer to Question 17

a) Maculopapular presentation of meningococcaemia.
b) Recent reports fail to substantiate claims of improved prognosis compared to the usual picture.

- Previously, a maculopapular presentation was considered to indicate an improved prognosis and a milder clinical course.
- As the macular rash may progress to haemorrhagic purpura, regular review is necessary.
- In one study of children with meningococcal septicaemia, 38% presented with maculopapular rashes with or without petechiae, whilst 13% had maculopapular rashes alone.

Marzouk O, Thomsen A P J, Sills J A et al 1991. Features and outcome in meningococcal disease presenting with a maculopapular rash. Arch. Dis. Child. 66:485–487

Question 18

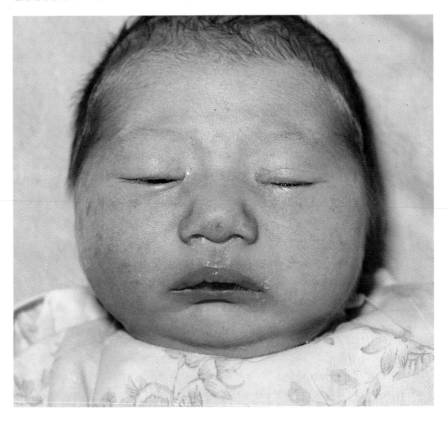

a) What is the diagnosis in this 46XY child?
b) List four associated features.
c) What is the significance of seeking an auditory assessment?

Answer to Question 18

a) Congenital hypothyroidism

b) Myxoedematous macroglossia; hoarse cry, hypotonia, umbilical hernia, constipation, prolonged neonatal unconjugated hyper-bilirubinaemia, transient or recurrent hypothermia, enlarged (>1 cm) posterior fontanelle and bradycardia

c) Pendred syndrome (incidence 2:100 000)

- Incidence 1:4000–6000.
- Female preponderance quoted for thyroid dysgenesis.
- About 5% of cases manifest clinical abnormalities in first week of life.
- More common in Down syndrome (1:128).
- Thyroid dysgenesis > dyshormonogenesis (10%).
- Infants more commonly exhibit post-term gestation and birth weight >3500 g.
- Pronounced skin mottling may occur (cutis marmorata).
- Plasma T4 levels at diagnosis <30 mmol/l are more likely to be associated with agenesis and more severe clinical features.
- Prolonged jaundice arises from impaired bilirubin excretion and increased enterohepatic circulation.
- ECG may show low voltage and prolonged conduction time.
- Delayed ossification occurs; particularly seen in the knee. Excessive thyroxine replacement can cause craniosynostosis.

Fisher D A 1989 Congenital hypothyroidism. In: Brook C (ed) Clinical paediatric endocrinology, 2nd edn. Blackwell Scientific Publications, Oxford
Grant D B, Smith I, Fuggle P W et al 1992 Congenital hypothyroidism detected by neonatal screening: relationship between biochemical severity and early clinical features. Arch. Dis. Child. 67:87–91

Question 19

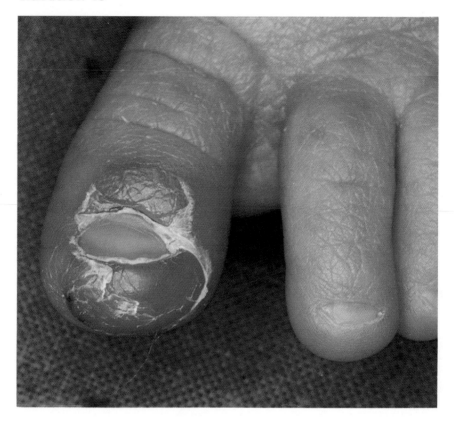

This infant was referred with poor feeding and irritability.

a) What is the diagnosis?
b) What is the most likely causative organism?
c) List four other types of sepsis caused by this organism.

Answer to Question 19

a) Cellulitis resulting from a paronychial infection
b) Staphylococcus aureus
c) Omphalitis
Osteomyelitis
Septicaemia
Pneumonia
Toxic epidermal necrolysis (Lyell or Ritter disease)

- Toxic epidermal necrolysis is potentially life-threatening due to exotoxin producing phage types (usually group II types 55 or 71).
- Skin friction causes epidermal shearing (Nikolsky sign).
- Parenteral antistaphylococcal antibiotics are required.

Question 20

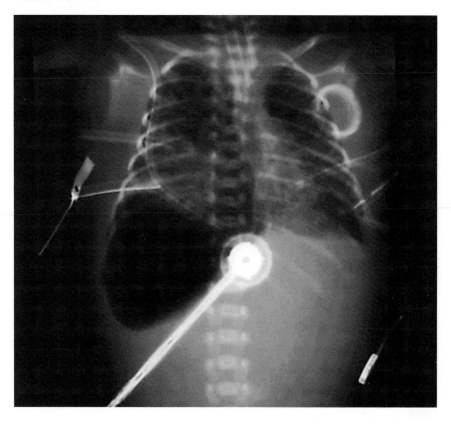

A preterm infant of 29 weeks' gestation became acidotic and hypotensive during ventilation for hyaline membrane disease. This is the emergency chest radiograph.

a) What is the cause of the sudden deterioration?
b) How would you try to prevent such an occurrence?
c) What neurological sequelae may ensue?

Answer to Question 20

a) Right tension pneumothorax. There is evidence of previous pneumothoraces and indwelling chest drains.

b) Ventilator manipulation to avoid long inspiratory times. Avoidance of high peak inspiratory pressures. Avoidance of active expiration asynchronously with the ventilator cycle. This may be achieved by increasing the ventilator rate to capture the infant's natural respiratory rate or by sedation and artificial paralysis.

c) Periventricular haemorrhage.

- Pneumothoraces occur in up to 35% of very low birth weight infants. They may occur in response to high intrapulmonary pressures due to the ventilator or active expiration against the ventilator cycle.
- Paralysis or sedation may prevent some pneumothoraces.
- The risk of pneumothoraces increases in the presence of pulmonary interstitial emphysema. The development of air leaks is associated with increased secretion of vasopressin which may lead to hyponatraemia.
- Systemic hypotension resulting from pneumothoraces may lead to cerebral hypoperfusion and cerebral injury. Haemorrhage may occur once the circulating volume and cerebral perfusion are restored.
- The effect of exogenous surfactant upon the incidence of pneumothoraces is still uncertain although some studies suggest a reduction in their occurrence.

Greenough A, Morley C J, Davis J A et al 1984 Pancuronium prevents pneumothoraces in ventilated premature babies who actively expire against positive pressure inflation. Lancet i:1–3
Lipscomb A P, Thornburn R J, Reynolds E O R et al 1981 Pneumothorax and cerebral haemorrhage in preterm infants. Lancet i:414–416
Morley C J 1991 Surfactant treatment for premature babies. Arch. Dis. Child. 66:445–450

Question 21

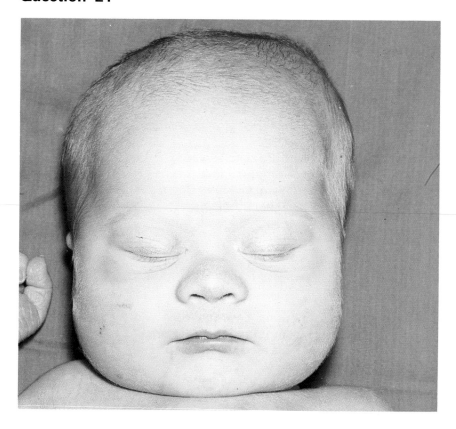

a) What is the diagnosis?
b) List five characteristic facial features of your diagnosis.
c) Give three potential problems encountered in the neonatal period.

Answer to Question 21

a) Down syndrome
b) Brachycephaly, microcephaly, slanted palpebral fissures, epicanthic folds, Brushfield spots, glossoptosis, small nose with widened nasal bridge, small ears with cartilaginous defects, microstomia and cataracts
c) Congenital cardiac disease
Duodenal atresia and other GI atresia or stenosis
Cataracts
Poor feeding and unco-ordinated sucking
Constipation due to poor fluid intake
Congenital hypothyroidism (1:300 of Down sufferers)
Parental anxiety, emotional problems, etc.

- Congenital cardiac defects in 20–40%; classically A-V canal defects in 50%.
- Routine echocardiography is recommended. Cardiac disease is responsible for 35% of deaths and mortality is highest in those under 2 years of age.
- 5% have GI malformations. Constipation is very common.
- Skin problems are common: 75% have areas of hyperkeratosis; seborrhoeic dermatitis is recognized and pronounced skin mottling (cutis marmorata) occurs.
- Up to 50% have cataracts in the neonatal period. Hypermetropia and defective nasolacrimal duct canalization are common. Myopia is present in about 20%.
- Sleep apnoea due to upper airways obstruction is common. There is increased susceptibility to middle ear infections; over 50% of children have hearing deficits.

Newton R W, Newton J A 1992 The management of Down's syndrome. In: David T J (ed) Recent advances in paediatrics, Vol 10. Churchill Livingstone, Edinburgh

Question 22

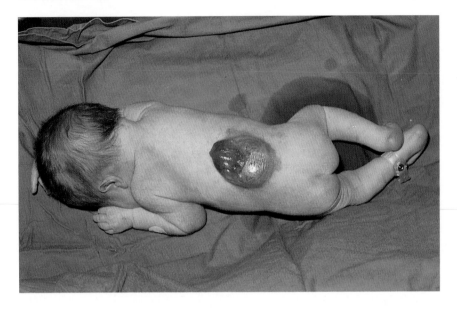

This infant has a meningomyelocele.

a) Give four potential problems encountered by this infant.
b) List five features considered to impart a poor prognosis when a pre-operative assessment is performed.
c) How may such a defect be detected antenatally?

Answer to Question 22

a) Urinary retention with overflow
Nephropathy due to high pressure vesico-ureteric reflux
Constipation with faecal overflow
Spastic diplegia
Hydrocephalus
Meningitis
b) Thoracolumbar lesion
Severe paraplegia
Kyphoscoliosis
Hydrocephalus
Intracerebral birth injury
Severe co-existing congenital defect
c) Elevated maternal serum alphafetoprotein level with subsequent elevated amniotic alphafetoprotein levels
Detailed anomaly scan

- Incidence 0.5–4:1000 live births.
- Reduction in incidence in 'at risk' pregnancies following first trimester vitamin B complex and folic acid administration.
- 80% develop hydrocephalus requiring treatment.
- Arnold–Chiari malformation may co-exist.
- Intermittent catheterization is regarded as the best method or urinary control. Renal function and the presence of reflux must be monitored.
- 70% of sufferers walk to some degree eventually.
- Orthopaedic surveillance is necessary to detect spinal instability or scoliosis.

Lorber J 1973 Early results of selective treatment of spina bifida cystica. Br. Med. J. IV:201–204

Question 23

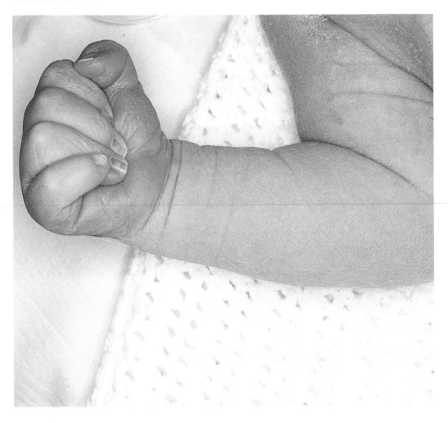

a) What dysmorphic feature is shown?
b) What is the most likely diagnosis?
c) List four other features.

Answer to Question 23

a) Clenched hand with overlapping fifth finger
b) Edward syndrome
c) Micrognathia
   Occipital prominence
   Low set malformed ears
   Rockerbottom feet
   Short sternum
   Cryptorchidism

- Incidence 1:6000 live births.
- <10% survive one year.
- Long term survivors are usually mosaics.
- 90% have cardiac defects.
- Renal defects are common.
- Risk increases with maternal age.

Question 24

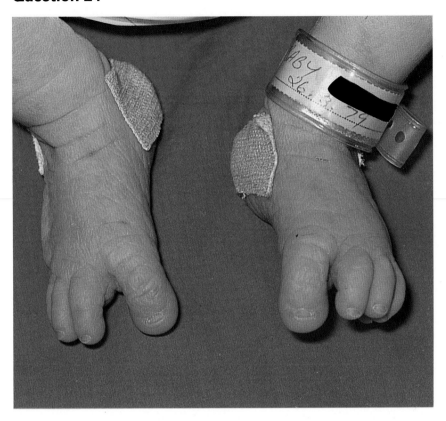

a) What is the most likely diagnosis?
b) Comment upon the likely growth pattern of this child.
c) Give three conditions known to be more prevalent in those with this condition.

Answer to Question 24

a) Wide gap between 1st and 2nd toes–Down syndrome
b) Reduced growth and resultant short stature. Delayed skeletal ossification
c) Alzheimer's disease
Epilepsy
Leukaemia
Hypothyroidism
Auto-immune diseases, e.g. vitiligo
Alopecia areata and totalis

- Growth retardation occurs leading to short stature. IGF-1 levels are low. There are some reports of response to high doses of exogenous growth hormone but although the height velocity is increased, the effect on final height is not yet known.
- 5% of adolescents have biochemical indices of hypothyroidism. 25% of adults have antithyroid antibodies with clinical manifestation in 15–17%. TSH levels tend to increase with age.
- Atlanto-axial dislocation is rare.
- IQ is variable: scores are higher in mosaics; scores tend to decrease with age and 13% have behavioural problems. Many attain a reading age of between 8 and 12 years.
- The incidence of leukaemia is higher than the general population. The remission rate is lower (81%) and the induction mortality is greater (14%). This may be due to greater susceptibility to sepsis and myelotoxicity.
- Other 'feet' cases in the MRCP examination include:
Turner syndrome
Rubinstein–Taybi syndrome
Apert syndrome
Toe clubbing
Edward syndrome
Patau syndrome
Keratoderma blenorrhagica.

Question 25

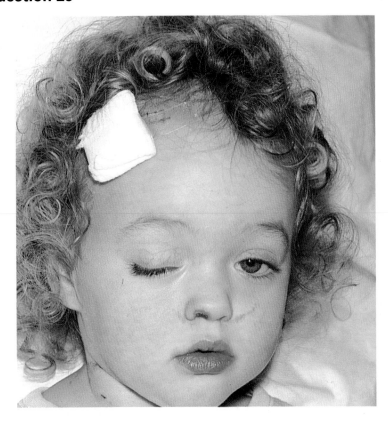

This girl is recovering from pneumococcal meningitis.

a) Describe the physical sign demonstrated.
b) List four potential complications of bacterial meningitis.
c) What prophylaxis should be offered to this child's family?

Answer to Question 25

a) Right third cranial nerve palsy: complete ptosis, divergent strabismus with the eye 'down and out' and pupillary dilatation (not shown).

b) Seizures (acute or chronic)
Cranial nerve palsies
Deafness
Cerebral infarction, abscess or cerebral palsy
Ophthalmitis
Hydrocephalus (usually communicating)
Subdural effusion
Syndrome of inappropriate ADH secretion
Adrenal haemorrhage (Waterhouse–Friedreichsen syndrome)
Endocarditis

c) None. Prophylaxis required for haemophilus and meningococcal meningitis. *Rifampicin*

- Pneumococcal meningitis is a serious and notifiable disease. Mortality reaches 15% with major neurological sequelae in 25% of survivors.
- There may be a pre-existing focus of infection. Bacteraemia is almost invariable.
- Blood cultures are usually positive. Latex agglutination test is positive in 50–75% of cases.
- Treatment is traditionally continued for 10 days.
- Dexamethasone may reduce mortality and long term morbidity, particularly deafness, in pneumococcal meningitis. Reduction in deafness but not mortality has been suggested in those with haemophilus meningitis. The greatest benefit may be seen if the dexamethasone is given before or at the time of antibiotic administration.
- Endocarditis is a rare, and often fatal, complication. Normal valves may be affected.

Levin M 1991 Bacterial meningitis. In: David T J (ed) Recent advances in paediatrics, Vol 9. Churchill Livingstone, Edinburgh

Question 26

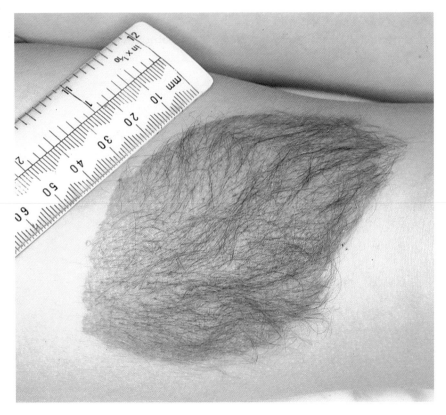

a) What is the diagnosis?
b) What is your management?

Answer to Question 26

a) Giant hairy naevus.
b) Remains debated. Many advise surgical removal to reduce the risk of melanomatous transformation.

- Giant hairy naevi may become malignant in up to 30%.
- They are an abnormality of dermal melanocytes.
- Some are extensive–'bathing trunk' naevi.
- Surgical removal may require skin grafting. Regular review is mandatory.

Question 27

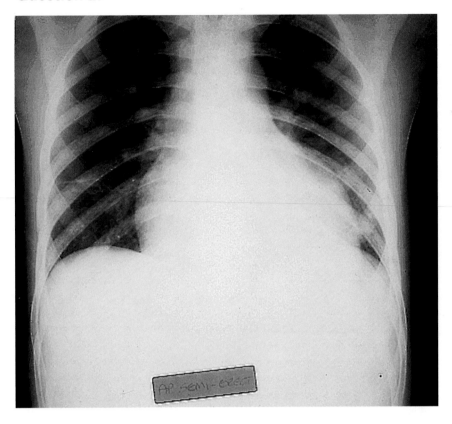

A teenage boy with homozygous sickle cell disease presented with breathlessness, tachycardia, hepatomegaly and a long systolic murmur. He had received multiple blood transfusions in the past. This is his chest radiograph.

a) What is the most significant radiological feature?
b) What is the most likely diagnosis? Give two possible causes.
c) List two helpful investigations to confirm your diagnosis.

Answer to Question 27

a) Cardiomegaly
b) Cardiac failure
Possible aetiologies: haemosiderotic cadiomyopathy
                       endocarditis due to immunosuppression
                       myocarditis
c) Echocardiography
ECG
Cardiac radionuclide scans
Ferritin and iron store studies
Septic screen

- Repeated transfusions may result in iron overload leading to cardiomyopathy and arrhythmias (particularly supraventricular arrhythmias).
- Haemosiderosis is prevented by the avoidance of repeated transfusions and the use of desferrioxamine chelation if such therapy is unavoidable.
- Transfusions may be given for aplastic crises but there is little evidence of amelioration of acute painful crises. Exchange transfusions are preferable when HbSS levels need reduction pre-operatively or following neurological and respiratory crises.
- Features of iron overload include: poor growth, delayed puberty, hypoparathyroidism, adrenal insufficiency, hepatosplenomegaly, arthropathy and late diabetes mellitus.
- Desferrioxamine therapy predisposes to yersinia infection. Repeated transfusions increases the risk of hepatitis C infection which is associated with a moderate mortality and high risk of chronic liver disease.

Ortega J A 1982 Clinical consequences and management of chronic iron overload. In: Willoughby M, Siegel S E (eds) Haematology and oncology (paediatrics 1). Butterworths, London

Question 28

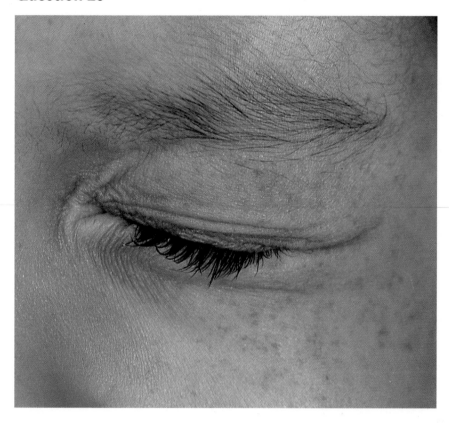

This child has been held by the neck by friends and exhibits a play-associated injury.

a) What physical sign is demonstrated?
b) What is the pathophysiology?
c) Give two occasions when this sign is also seen.

Answer to Question 28

a) Peri-orbital petechiae.

b) Obstruction to the venous drainage of the head, associated with a degree of hypoxia due to tracheal compression, causing capillary rupture.

c) Pertussis (following a coughing spasm)

Non-accidental injury

Parturition (when the umbilical cord is wrapped around the infant's neck).

- This injury may be accompanied by subconjunctival haemorrhages.
- Retinal haemorrhage must be excluded. These are commonly but not exclusively seen in abuse cases.
- Play-associated injuries may mimic and be mistaken for child abuse. Such injuries have been associated with television viewing habits.
- Traumatic peri-orbital petechiae were first described by the French police surgeon Tardieu.

Gadow K D, Sprafkin J 1989 Television violence. Paediatrics 83:399–405

Question 29

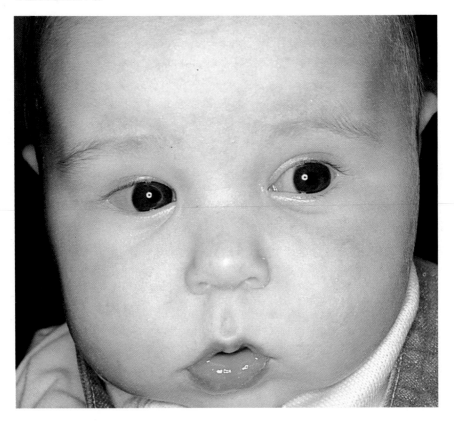

This infant has a humeral fracture.

a) What is the underlying diagnosis?
b) What is the aetiology of this diagnosis?
c) What may be seen on the skull radiograph?

Answer to Question 29

a) Osteogenesis imperfecta
b) Heterogeneous group of disorders of Type I collagen synthesis
c) Wormian bones (often occipital)
    Previous fractures

- Variable inheritance 1:10 000–50 000; 80% of cases are Type I.
- Severity of the disease tends to be similar within one family.
- Inheritance: dominant in I and IV; recessive (usually) in II and III.
- Type II is often lethal in the perinatal period. Bones are short, broad and deformed.
- Blue sclerae with premature arcus may be absent in Types III and IV.
- Dentinogenesis imperfecta with translucent teeth is associated.
- Deafness (>50% by 50 years) is common. Otosclerosis is also commonly detected.
- Other evidence of collagen disease includes: joint hypermobility, tendon rupture and aortic valve regurgitation.
- Diaphyseal fractures are more common than metaphyseal lesions.
- Genetic abnormalities on chromosomes 7 and 17. The defect seems to be overhydroxylation of alpha 1 (I) chain collagen.
- Antenatal diagnosis is available; mild disease may be detected in asymptomatic family members by the presence of Wormian bones on plain skull radiographs.

Smith R 1984 Osteogenesis imperfecta. Br. Med. J. 289:394–395

Question 30

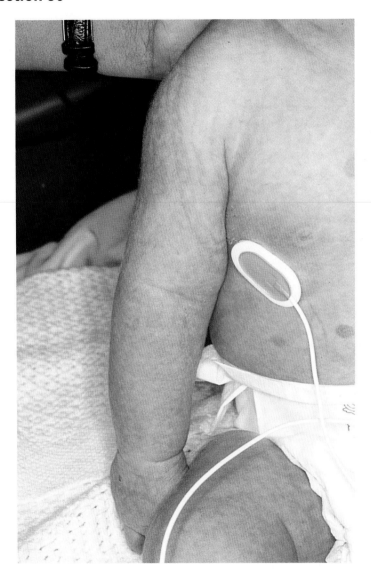

a) What abnormality is shown?
b) What is the likely prognosis?

Answer to Question 30

a) Right Erb palsy
b) Full recovery in most cases

- Erb palsy is a neuropraxia of C5/C6 roots of the brachial plexus. The arm is limp and rests in pronation.
- The other main brachial plexus injury is Klumpke palsy.
- Pseudoparalysis is noted on examination with an absent Moro reflex. Fractures of the clavicle and humerus may co-exist.
- Predisposing factors include: breech delivery, shoulder dystocia and macrosomia.

Question 31

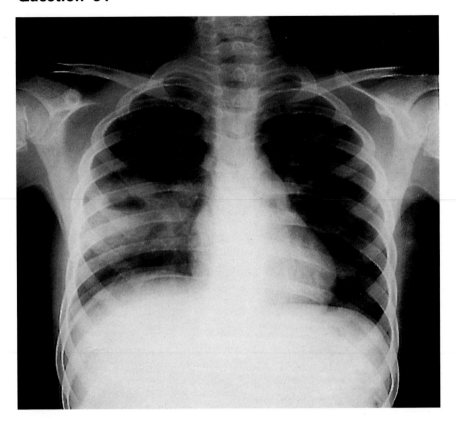

a) What is the diagnosis?
b) List three potential causative organisms.
c) List four recognized complications of your diagnosis.

Answer to Question 31

a) Right middle lobe pulmonary abscess
b) Pneumococcus
   Staphylococcus
   Haemophilus influenzae
   Klebsiella pneumoniae
   Mycobacterium tuberculosis
   Mycotic infections
   Entamoeba histolytica
   Anaerobes
   Legionella
c) Bronchiectasis
   Bronchial stenosis
   Haemorrhage
   Bronchopleural fistula and empyema
   Secondary sepsis including cerebral abscess
   Mediastinitis
   Osteo-arthropathy

- Right lung is more commonly affected. Predisposing factors include aspiration of foreign bodies, cysts, poor oral hygiene and immuno-suppression.
- Haemoptysis is common. Micro-abscesses are more common in cystic fibrosis than large abscesses. Clubbing may develop.
- Failure of resolution indicates the need for bronchoscopy. Recurrence may be due to ciliary dyskinesia or Kartagener syndrome.
- Residual defects, not detected on plain X-ray, may be seen on ventilation/perfusion isotope scanning.

O'Callaghan C 1989 Paediatric radiology. Wolfe, London

Question 32

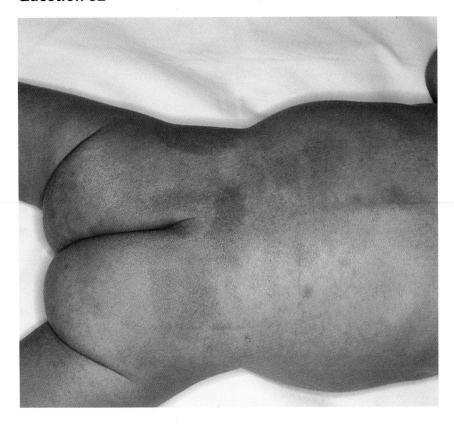

This picture was obtained at a routine 6 week infant examination.

a) What is demonstrated?
b) What investigations would you perform? What is the management?

Answer to Question 32

a) Mongolian blue spot
b) None. Reassure the parents

- Histologically, these are dermal melanocytic naevi.
- Their classic site is over the sacrum.
- Whilst some may persist, most fade between the ages of 4 and 7 years.
- There is a higher frequency in the Asian population. They occur in 10% of white children.

Question 33

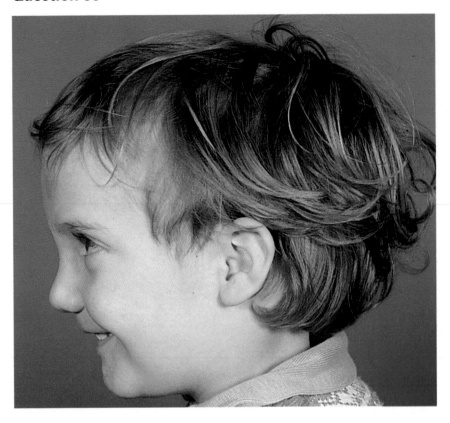

a) What abnormality is illustrated?
b) What is the cause of the abnormality?
c) List three possible complications encountered as a result of this diagnosis.

Answer to Question 33

a) Abnormal head shape–craniosynostosis. Scaphocephaly in this case.
b) Premature fusion of the skull sutures. The sagittal sutures are affected in scaphocephaly.
c) Increased intracranial pressure (rare in scaphocephaly)
   Exophthalmos
   Cranial nerve palsies
   Strabismus
   Deafness
   Cosmetic concerns.

- Craniosynostosis may be an isolated problem or part of a syndrome, e.g. Apert.
- It is an acquired defect in hypophosphatasia and severe rickets.
- Achondroplasia may mimic scaphocephaly due to an imbalance of endochondral and membranous ossification, particularly in the basal bones, giving rise to the characteristic head shape seen in this condition.
- Overtreated congenital hypothyroidism has been associated with premature suture fusion.
- The management of craniosynostosis requires a multidisciplinary team approach.

Hayward R 1990 Craniosynostosis and the paediatrician. Arch. Dis. Child. 65:568–569

Question 34

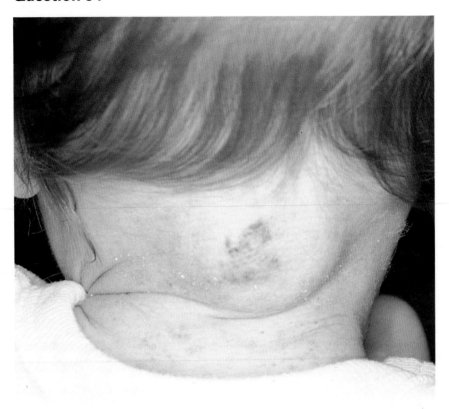

a) What is the diagnosis?
b) Give two potential complications.

Answer to Question 34

a) Posterior cervical cavernous haemangioma
b) Ulceration
   Haemorrhage
   Sepsis
   Pressure effects on deeper structures

- Haemangiomata are benign lesions. Multiple internal haemangio-mata may co-exist.
- Surgical excision may be hazardous. Steroids may aid regression if these lesions are problematic.
- Massive multiple internal haemangiomata may cause high-output cardiac failure and require embolization.
- Thrombocytopenia due to platelet sequestration and consumption within giant haemangiomata (Kasabach–Merritt syndrome) occurs in conjuction with disseminated intravascular coagulation.
- Therapeutic options include: radiotherapy, tranexamic acid, aspirin and, if a limb is affected, external compression.
- Limb haemangiomata may be associated with asymmetrical limb growth (Klippel–Trenaunay–Weber syndrome).

Aylett S E, Williams A F, Brown D H 1990 The Kasabach–Merritt syndrome: treatment with intermittent pneumatic compression. Arch. Dis. Child. 65:790–792

Question 35

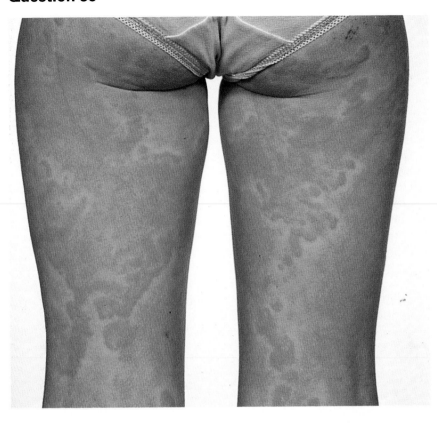

This child was brought to the Accident and Emergency Department with difficulty in breathing following the ingestion of strawberries. Examination revealed this rash and acute stridor.

a) What is the diagnosis?
b) What is your emergency management?

Answer to Question 35

a) Angio-oedema with urticaria

b) Intravenous administration of hydrocortisone and antihistamine
Intramuscular adrenaline
Airway management if upper airway obstruction persists.

- Many foodstuffs may cause urticaria and angio-oedema.
- Angio-oedema affects the subcutaneous tissue and is often painful; urticaria is pruritic and affects the upper dermis.
- Urticaria is IgE mediated. Chronic cases (>2 months) may be due to an identifiable cause in 20%.
- Urticaria is associated with: SLE, malignancy, thyroid disease and IgG subclass deficiency.
- Hereditary angio-oedema may result from C1 esterase inhibitor deficiency which is an autosomal dominant inheritance in many cases. Serum C4 is invariably low. It may rarely present as recurrent stridor.
- C1 esterase deficiency may respond to danazol or tranexamic acid. Danazol increases C1 inhibitor production whereas tranexamic acid inhibits plasmin which consumes C1 inhibitor.
- Thyroid auto-antibodies are 3–7 times more common in females with angio-oedema.

Watson J G, Bird A G 1990 Urticaria and angioedema. In: Watson J G, Bird A G (eds) Handbook of immunological investigations in children. Wright, London

Question 36

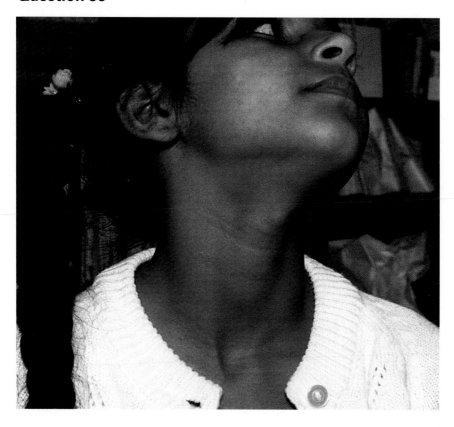

A small anterior mass was noted on routine examination of this teenager's neck.

a) What is the most likely diagnosis?
b) By what simple test can the diagnosis be confirmed?
c) What is the treatment?

Answer to Question 36

a) Thyroglossal cyst
b) Movement of the mass when the tongue is protruded or the patient swallows
c) Surgical excision of the cyst and its tract

- Thyroglossal cysts result from a failure of obliteration of the embryonic thyroglossal duct.
- They may occur anywhere along a line from the glossal foramen caecum to the thyroid isthmus.
- Sepsis and haemorrhage are two rare complications.
- Prior to surgery, the cyst must be differentiated from an ectopic thyroid gland. Removal involves the excision of the mid-portion of the hyoid bone (Sistrunk operation).

Question 37

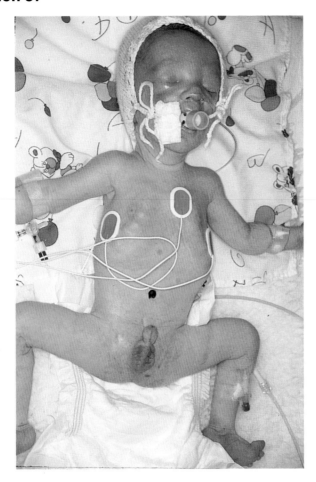

This term neonate requires mechanical ventilation. He is neither sedated nor pharmacologically paralysed.

a) Comment upon this infant's posture.
b) List four possible diagnoses.
c) Give four useful investigations to aid your diagnosis.

Answer to Question 37

a) 'Froglike' posture suggesting marked hypotonia

b) There are many aetiologies including:

Birth asphyxia; Werdnig–Hoffman disease (severe spinal muscular atrophy); congenital myopathy (myotubular, central core and, occasionally, nemaline types); myotonic dystrophy; congenital myasthenia; chromosomal abnormalities (Prader–Willi syndrome, etc.); cerebral palsy; cervical cord trauma; metabolic disorders and mitochondrial cytopathies

c) Investigations include:

Electromyography (EMG)
Muscle enzymes, e.g. creatine kinase
Muscle biopsy
Nerve conduction studies
Cranial ultrasound
Edrophonium (Tensilon) test
Karyotype
ECG
Sural nerve biopsy
Metabolic studies

- Antenatal polyhydramnios may herald myotonic dystrophy.
- Features of myotonic dystrophy include facial diplegia with 'fish mouth' facies and a poor sucking reflex. Genetic markers used in diagnosis are linked on chromosome 19.
- An elevated serum creatine kinase within the first 10 days of life is of dubious significance.
- Werdnig–Hoffman disease is associated with glossal fasciculation. The EMG may be normal but the muscle action potential is usually reduced.

Question 38

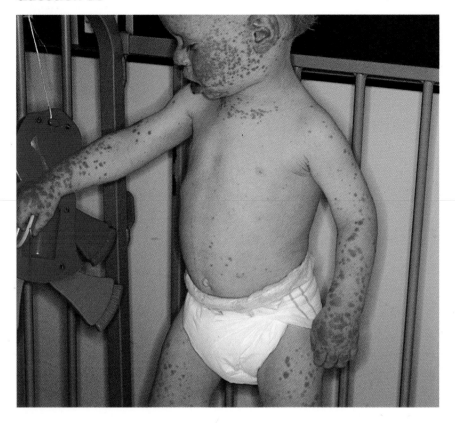

The rash shown above was noted in a well child after a picnic.

a) What is the diagnosis?
b) Give one aetiology.

Answer to Question 38

a) Phytophotodermatitis
b) Giant hogweed plant

- The distribution is classical–occurring peripherally on exposed areas of skin.
- The rash may be florid and cause great concern to all except the child who is rarely disturbed by it.
- Many plants may be responsible for these reactions.
- Residual pigmentary changes occur.
- Disorders exacerbated by light include: herpes simplex, psoriasis, SLE and Darier disease.

Question 39

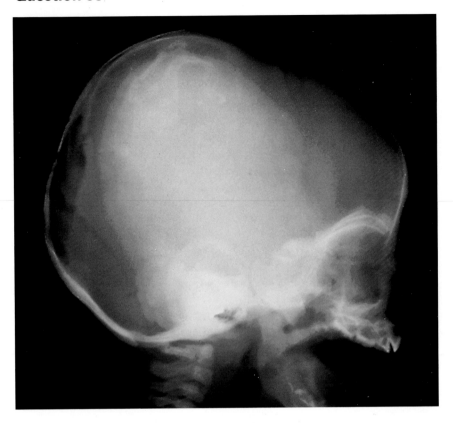

This is a skull radiograph of an asymptomatic infant.

a) What is the radiological abnormality?
b) List three complications of this diagnosis in the neonatal period.
c) What is your management?

Answer to Question 39

a) Calcified right parietal cephalhaematoma
b) Neonatal unconjugated hyperbilirubinaemia
Infection leading to skulll osteomyelitis
Ulceration of overlying scalp
Cosmetic concerns and parental anxieties
c) None. Reassure parents

- The cephalhaematoma is a subperiosteal haemorrhage. Its extension is therefore limited by the sutures. They may arise spontaneously or after documented instrumental or difficult deliveries.
- They differ from caput succadenaeum and post-Ventouse chignon which are soft tissue oedematous swellings.
- Differentiation from the more serious, and potentially extensive, subaponeurotic haemorrhage which is not limited by sutures. Hypovolaemia, shock and anaemia are potential complications.
- Resolution of the cephalhaematoma is usually complete although calcification can occur.
- Severe intracephalhaematoma erythrocyte lysis may result in unconjugated hyperbilirubinaemia requiring phototherapy.

Question 40

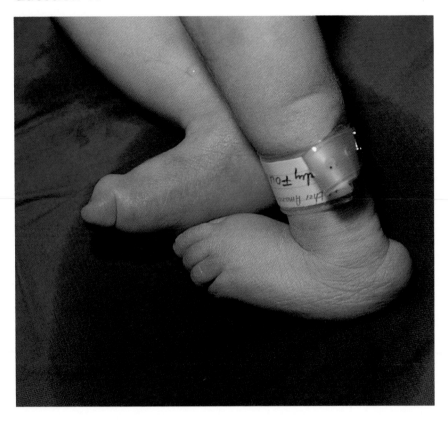

a) What dysmorphic feature is demonstrated?
b) Give two clinical diagnoses.
c) List three associated abnormalities of your diagnosis.

Answer to Question 40

a) Rockerbottom feet
b) Patau syndrome (trisomy 13)
   Edward syndrome (trisomy 18) (see Question 23)
c) Cleft lip +/− cleft palate
   Coloboma
   Cataracts
   Microphthalmia
   Broad nose
   Low set ears
   Scalp defects
   Post-axial polydactyly
   Cardiac and renal defects

- Patau syndrome incidence 1:8000.
- Described in 1960.
- 80% mortality in the first year.
- 80% have cardiac defects.
- 60% have renal defects.
- There is a wide range of cerebral malformations. Risk increases with increasing maternal age.

Question 41

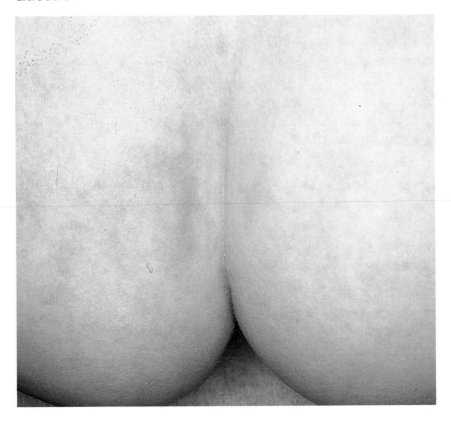

A child was admitted with a skull fracture following a fall at home. A nurse noted this appearance of the buttocks whilst changing her nappy.

a) Describe the appearance. What may have caused this?
b) Briefly outline your further management.

Answer to Question 41

a) Horseshoe punctate lesion arising on the left buttock. Human bite-mark

b) History and examination including fundoscopy
Discussion with a senior colleague
Interview family members and those witness to the fall
Contact Child Protection Team
Clotting profile and platelet count
Clinical photography
Consider skeletal survey to exclude other current and historical injury

- Adults do bite children as a form of abuse!
- Clues to abuse from the history include:
  Delay in presentation to health teams
  Vague and often inconsistent history
  Interperson variation in story
  Abnormal parental affect
  Abnormal child behaviour, e.g. frozen watchfulness
  Different account of the injury from the child.
- Radiological features suggestive of abuse include:
  Multiple fractures of differing ages
  Metaphyseal–epiphyseal fractures ('bucket-handle')
  Rib fractures (particularly posterior ribs)
  Spiral long bone fractures
  Single wide skull fractures with multiple bruises
  Multiple or wide complex skull fractures.
- Deliberate burning accounts for 10% of cases.
- Sexual abuse may co-exist; anal abuse occurs in both sexes.
  Sexually transmitted diseases must be excluded if sexual abuse has occurred.

Meadow R 1986 ABC of child abuse. BMJ Publications, London

Question 42

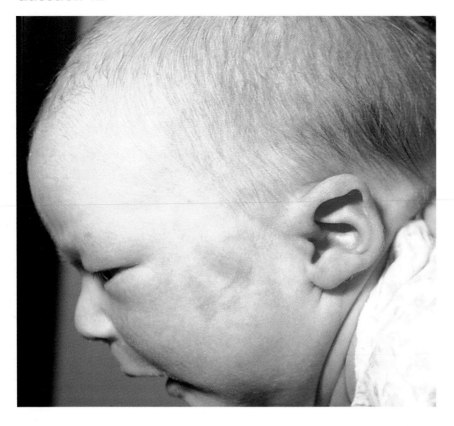

a) What dysmorphic feature is demonstrated?
b) Give two associated diagnoses.

Answer to Question 42

a) Low set ears
b) Potter syndrome
   Patau syndrome
   Edward syndrome
   Turner syndrome

- Potter syndrome: renal agenesis, pulmonary hypoplasia and limb contractures.
- Antenatal clue to diagnosis is the presence of oligohydramnios.
- Low set ears are seen in up to 80% of those with Turner syndrome.

Question 43

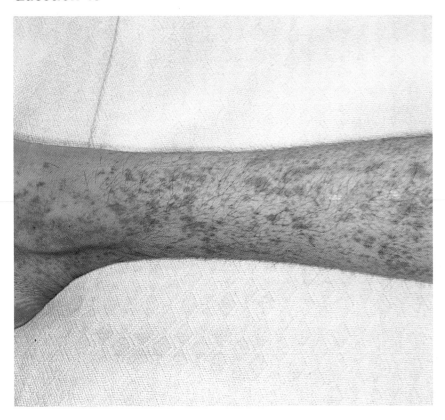

This boy was admitted with a rash and a recent history of severe epistaxis. He was unwell with symptoms of an upper respiratory tract infection. He had taken aspirin and quinine because of his symptoms. The quinine belonged to his father who always took them for muscular pains associated with 'flu. There was no family history of bleeding disorders.

a) What is the cause of the rash? Give two possible causes.
b) List three investigations to confirm your diagnosis.

Answer to Question 43

a) Thrombocytopenic purpura

Idiopathic thrombocytopenic purpura (ITP)
Viral induced thrombocytopenia
Drug induced thrombocytopenia (both aspirin and quinine)
Aplastic anaemia
Underlying leukaemia
b) Blood count and film
Coagulation profile and factor assays (if indicated)
Bleeding time
Bone marrow aspiration
Platelet function tests
Viral serology and septic screen
Drug–hapten estimation

- Aspirin may cause platelet dysfunction by irreversible inhibition of the cyclo-oxygenase system.
- Hypersensitivity to quinine, which may be recurrent, can cause thrombocytopenia.
- ITP may be preceded by a viral illness and is usually self-limiting. Antiglycoprotein antibodies may be the best guide to prognosis and the development of chronic ITP.
- Congenital platelet abnormalities may present acutely. Glanzmann thrombasthenia may be cured by bone marrow transplantation in those who are platelet transfusion dependent.

Stevens R F 1989 The purpuras. In: Stevens R F (ed) Handbook of haematological investigations in children. Wright, London

Question 44

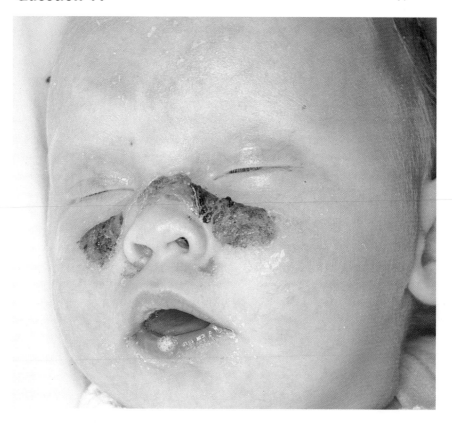

This infant became acutely unwell several days after exposure to the sun. She was collapsed, hypotensive with profuse diarrhoea and peripheral desquamation. This picture, taken during convalescence, shows the last remnants of the underlying, preceding problem.

a) What was the underlying problem?
b) What was the cause of the subsequent collapse?
c) List the relevant criteria for the establishment of the diagnosis.

Answer to Question 44

a) Impetiginous infection of sunburn (photo-erythema) as shown in the picture
b) Staphylococcal toxic shock syndrome (TTS)
c) Fever of at least 38.9°C
Macular erythema–patchy or generalized leading to patchy desquamation
Hypotension
Toxic action on at least three systems including:
Diarrhoea or vomiting
Myalgia or raised creatine kinase activity
Reddened conjunctivae, oropharynx or vagina
Elevated creatinine or urea
Thrombocytopenia
Confusion/drowsiness without focal neurological signs

- Initially associated with menstruation and tampon use in USA. May result from toxins from trivial staphylococcal infection or colonization. 13% of cases are non-menstrual associated.
- Toxic shock syndrome toxin-1 (TSST-1) is a 22 kDa protein which may be detected in vitro and in vivo and is involved in the triggering of a cytokine cascade. This probably results from T cell activation following binding of the toxin to class II major histocompatibility complex receptors.
- Intensive care is required. Studies with antitoxin are in progress. Antistaphylococcal and inotropic drugs are used.
- Mortality approximates to 3–10%.
- Group A beta haemolytic streptococci (GABHS) cause a similar clinical picture but do not arise from colonization or trivial sepsis, rather requiring serious infection with bacteraemia.

Reingold A L, Shands K N, Dan B B et al 1982 Toxic shock syndrome not associated with menstruation. Lancet i:1–4
Torres-Martinez C, Mehta D, Butt A et al 1992 Streptococcus associated toxic shock. Arch. Dis. Child. 67:126–131
Williams G R 1990 The toxic shock syndrome. Br. Med. J. 300:960

Question 45

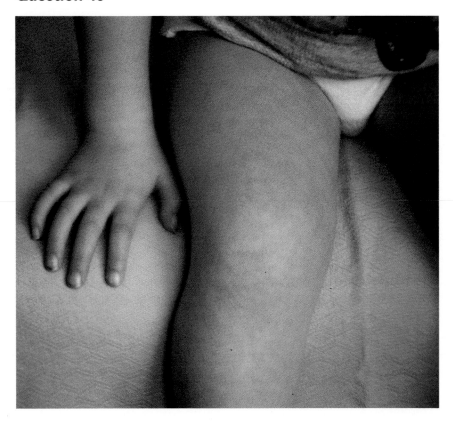

A 4-year-old girl presented with a history of recurrent swelling of her ankles and elbows for the last 6 months. On this admission, the above clinical feature was noted.

a) What is demonstrated in the above picture? Probable diagnosis?
b) Give four relevant investigations.
c) What treatment should be considered?

Answer to Question 45

a) Right knee swelling with probable effusion
Pauci-articular juvenile chronic arthritis (JCA)
b) Knee radiograph
Joint aspiration: cytology, microbiology and immunology
ESR and C-reactive protein (CRP)
Blood count and film
Auto-antibodies: rheumatoid factor, antinuclear (ANA), etc.
Ophthalmic assessment (slit lamp)
Immunoglobulin classes
Complement levels
Viral and atypical serology
Albumen: globulin ratio
c) Non-steroidal anti-inflammatory drugs, e.g. naproxen
Rest limb in the early stages, then physiotherapy
Topical ophthalmic steroids for uveitis

- Diagnosis of JCA: duration of symptoms >3 months, having commenced before the age of 16 years. Other diseases such as SLE must be excluded.
- Pauci-articular JCA occurs in 50–65% of cases. This type affects up to four joints, has a female preponderance (2:1) and usually presents before the age of 5 years. 70% of cases resolve by 16 years of age. There is rarely any destructive articular disease.
- The majority of patients have: elevated ESR (although this does not reliably reflect disease activity); normal CRP levels; elevated immunoglobulins and reversed albumin: globulin ratio.
- 4% of pauci-articular JCA patients have selective IgA deficiency.
- It is rheumatoid factor IgM negative. 50% have positive ANA. 80% of ANA positive patients develop uveitis, which is initially only detectable by slit lamp examination. 65% have bilateral involvement and usually, signs are detectable within 2 years of the onset of arthritis.
- Untreated eye disease may lead to cataracts and band keratopathy.

Craft A W 1985 The management of juvenile chronic arthritis. Br. J. Hosp. Med. 33:188–194

Question 46

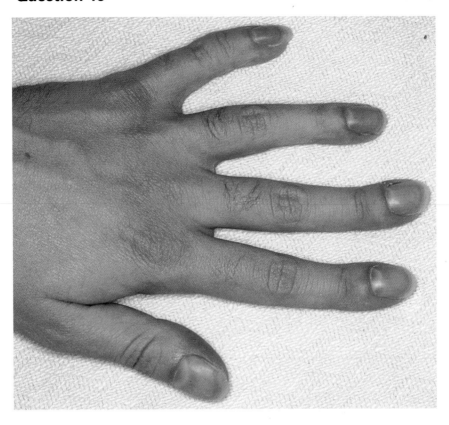

a) Describe two abnormalities seen in this picture.
b) List four causes for this appearance.

Answer to Question 46

a) Digital clubbing
Peripheral cyanosis
Clinodactyly (incidental finding in this case)
b) Cystic fibrosis
Bronchiectasis
Empyema and other chronic suppurative lung disease
Cyanotic cardiac disease
Inflammatory bowel disease
Rarely, subacute bacterial endocarditis

- Bronchiectasis comprises persistent dilatation of the bronchi with chronic sepsis. Major contributory factors include pneumonia, structural abnormalities and underlying disease such as cystic fibrosis, aspiration syndromes or foreign bodies.
- Pertussis may result in bronchiectasis. Convalescent chest X-rays are mandatory to exclude persistent lung collapse.
- Bronchiectasis may be visualized by plain radiography, CT scan, and ventilation/perfusion scan. Bronchography is advocated prior to surgery.
- Bronchiectasis is encountered in ciliary dyskinesia.

Buchdahl R M, Reiser J, Ingram D et al 1988 Ciliary abnormalities in respiratory disease. Arch. Dis. Child. 63:238–243
Dinwiddie R 1990 Respiratory tract infection. In: Dinwiddie R (ed) The diagnosis and management of paediatric respiratory disease. Churchill Livingstone, Edinburgh.

Question 47

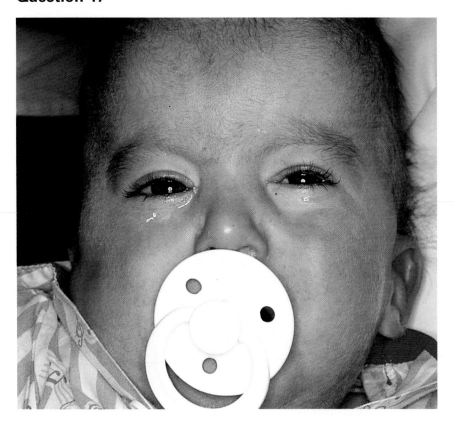

This child is dysmorphic. His anomalies failed to conform to a recognized pattern. Karyotyping revealed an unbalanced translocation from chromosome 7 to 10p.

a) Outline the general principles of management.
b) This child is re-admitted with recurrent apnoeic episodes. Give three possible causes and investigations to aid diagnosis.

Answer to Question 47

a) Mangement includes:
Exclusion of major system abnormalities, e.g. cardiac and GI
Screening for audiovisual defects
Genetic counselling
Guidance on feeding
Referral to the Child Development Team
Early educational assessment
Contact with parental support groups
Social service support
b) Seizures
Central apnoea
Obstructive apnoea
Infection, e.g. RSV bronchiolitis
Gastro-oesophageal reflux
EEG
Microlaryngoscopy
Oximetry and sleep studies
24 hour pH monitoring
CT brain scan
Infection screen

- The chromosomal abnormality caused: secundum atrioseptal defect; low set ears; pre-auricular pits; single palmar crease; micrognathia; bifid uvula; third fontanelle; developmental delay; upper airway obstruction; scoliosis and calcaneovalgus feet.
- Apnoea, due to upper airway obstruction, is common in many chromosomal defects.
- The association between apnoea and gastro-oesophageal reflux has been noted in many cases. Severe symptoms, not responding to medical measures, may require fundoplication.

Question 48

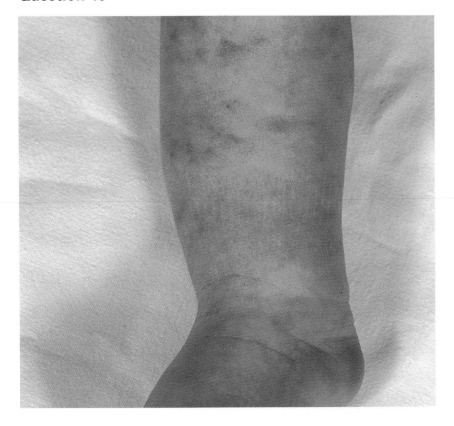

This infant was found, at home, collapsed and convulsing. He had been well throughout the preceding day. On admission, he was hypotensive and febrile with the above rash. He began bleeding from venepuncture sites and developed profuse bloody diarrhoea with subsequent renal and hepatic failure.

a) What is the cause of the skin appearance?
b) Give three differential diagnoses and four helpful investigations to aid your diagnosis.

Answer to Question 48

a) Skin ecchymoses and purpura
b) Differential diagnoses include:
Haemorrhagic shock and encephalopathy syndrome (HSE)
Toxic shock syndrome
Reye syndrome
Meningococcal septicaemia
Overwhelming viral infection, e.g. echo, adenovirus, etc.
Metabolic disease: urea cycle and MCAD defects
Heat shock/stroke
Rickettsial or leptospiral infection

c) Blood count and film
Coagulation studies
Electrolyte, glucose and acid-base studies
Renal and hepatic function tests
Muscle enzymes
Blood culture, septic screen, rapid antigen screen
Viral and atypical serology
Plasma ammonia
Serum immunoreactive trypsin/alpha-1-antitrypsin
Metabolic screen
Toxic shock syndrome toxin-1
EEG and CT brain scan

- HSE may have a sudden onset or a mild, non-specific prodrome. Vomiting is the presenting feature of the prodrome in 33%.
- Collapse and early coma occur. CT scans show oedema; haemorrhage, particularly into the pituitary gland, is seen at necropsy.
- There is usually a modest elevation of core temperature. No causative agent has yet been identified.
- Whilst similar to Reye syndrome, differentiation is possible. In Reye syndrome, ammonia levels are greatly elevated and profound hypoglycaemia occurs. Ammonia levels are normal or mildly elevated in HSE which is characterized by shock. Fatty hepatic infiltration is rare in HSE but invariable in Reye syndrome.
- Elevated immunoreactive trypsin and depressed alpha-1-antitrypsin occur in HSE and may be related to the pathogenesis of this condition. Whilst the outcome is poor, recent studies have shown normal development in some of the survivors.

Bacon C J, Hall S M 1992 Haemorrhagic shock encephalopathy syndrome in the British Isles. Arch. Dis. Child. 67:985–993
Levin M, Kay J D S, Gould J D et al 1983 Haemorrhagic shock and encephalopathy: a new syndrome with a high mortality in young children. Lancet ii: 64–67

Question 49

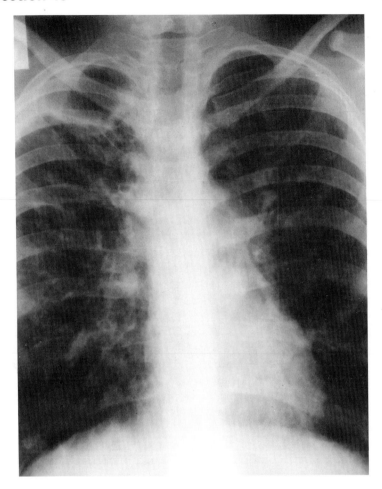

This is an X-ray of an adolescent with chronic respiratory symptoms.

a) What is the most likely diagnosis?
b) List four radiological features demonstrated on this X-ray.
c) Give two common cardiopulmonary complications.

Answer to Question 49

a) Cystic fibrosis
b) Bronchial wall thickening
   Mottled shadows (microlobular sputum retention)
   Hyperinflation
   Ring shadows (lobular bronchiectasis)
   Right apical bulla
c) Pneumothorax (20%)
   Haemoptysis (60%)
   Cor pulmonale
   Abscess
   Respiratory failure and death

- 50% of affected infants have respiratory symptoms by the age of 8 months.
- Pathological mechanisms include: recurrent sepsis, small airway obstruction, squamous metaplasia, mucus plugging, mucociliary disruption, micro-abscess formation and chronic bronchiectasis. Eventually, vascular shunting and vascular hypertrophy result in pulmonary hypertension.
- Progression of pulmonary disease may be monitored by scoring systems on plain radiography. One commonly used score is the Chrispin–Norman score; scores >20 indicate advanced disease.
- Over 50% wheeze. This may be due to: allergic reactions; asthma; bronchopulmonary aspergillosis and viral induced bronchial hyperresponsiveness. Aspergillosis is uncommon despite a positive skin test in 56% of children. However, bronchodilators and inhaled steroids may be of great benefit.
- Major respiratory pathogens include: staphylococci, haemophilus and, eventually, pseudomonas species. The latter is associated with a decline in respiratory function and, once present, is rarely eradicated. 60–90% of patients become chronically colonized.
- Pulmonary damage may be caused by free radicals and proteases produced by polymorphs and macrophages within the lung.

Chrispin A R, Norman A P 1974 The systematic evaluation of the chest radiograph in cystic fibrosis. Pediat. Radiol. 2:101–106
Dinwiddie R 1986 Management of the chest in CF. J. Roy. Soc. Med. 79 (Suppl. 12):6–9

Question 50

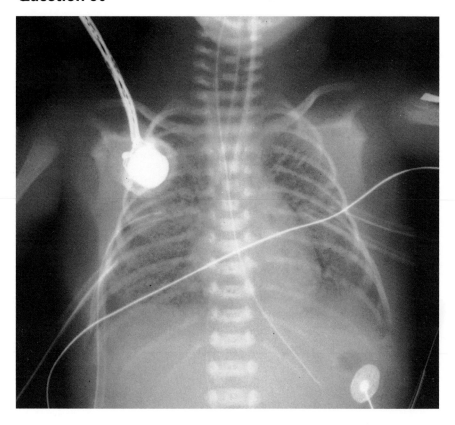

A preterm infant of 27 weeks' gestation remains ventilated at 5 weeks of age. This is the chest X-ray.

a) What is the likely diagnosis?
b) List three features on this X-ray consistent with your diagnosis.
c) Briefly outline your management.

Answer to Question 50

a) Bronchopulmonary dysplasia (BPD or chronic lung disease of the newborn)

b) Endotracheal intubated–indicating persistent ventilatory requirements

Cystic changes

Thickening of the bronchial walls

Diffuse reticular opacification with interstitial oedema

Chest drains indicating previous air leaks

c) Weaning from mechanical ventilation using short inspiratory times; trigger ventilation, etc.

Methylxanthines, e.g. caffeine or theophylline

Dexamethasone

Diuretics

Inhaled bronchodilators

Nutritional support

Avoidance and prompt treatment of sepsis including diseases such as RSV bronchiolitis

Continous negative pressure box

- Incidence of BPD varies from 4–70% depending upon the duration of ventilation and the gestation. BPD is generally defined as oxygen dependence in the presence of an abnormal chest X-ray after 28 days of postnatal age.
- Prophylaxis is avoidance of preterm deliveries. Reduction of barotrauma during prolonged ventilation and the avoidance of oxygen and free radical toxicity. These latter problems result in lipid peroxidation and membrane damage. Ethane and pentane, markers of peroxidation, are poor prognostic indicators.
- The use of free radical scavengers and anti-oxidants, such as vitamins A, C and E and superoxide dismutase, have been advocated.
- The effect of exogenous surfactant is still under evaluation.
- Steroids may be beneficial although there are side-effects such as GI bleeding and sepsis. Theophylline reduces the frequency and duration of respiratory pauses, reduces pulmonary artery pressure and improves diaphragmatic function. It has a synergistic action with diuretics.

Greenough A 1990 Bronchopulmonary dysplasia. Arch. Dis. Child. 65:1082–1088

Question 51

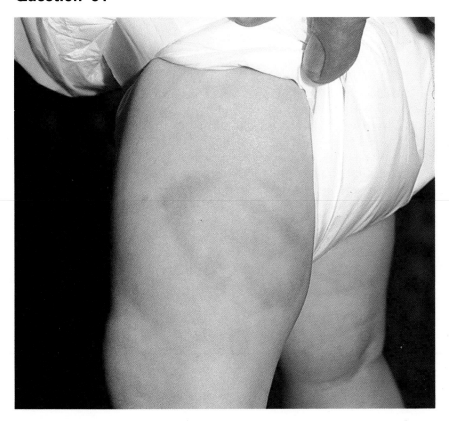

A 10-month-old boy was brought to clinic with a history of recent, unexplained bruising. Previous episodes had been noted by the health visitor. Haematological analysis revealed mild thrombocytopenia with large platelets seen on film. Clotting indices were normal except bleeding time.

a) Give a likely diagnosis and a confirmatory test.

Answer to Question 51

a) Bernard Soulier syndrome
Platelet aggregation studies: defective to ristocetin but not to ADP, adrenaline, collagen and arachidonic acid

- Rare autosomal disorder of purpura/bruising characterized by moderate thrombocytopenia and large platelets.
- Abnormality of platelet membrane glycoprotein I.
- Deficiency of the membrane receptor for ristocetin activity accounts for the abnormal aggregation studies.
- Glanzmann disease shows abnormal aggregation studies to ADP and collagen plus ristocetin in most cases.
- Large platelets are also seen in May–Hegglin anomaly whilst small platelets occur in the Wiskott–Aldrich syndrome. This has a sex-linked inheritance.

Stevens R F 1989. The purpuras. In: Stevens R F (ed) Handbook of haematological investigations in children. Wright, London

Question 52

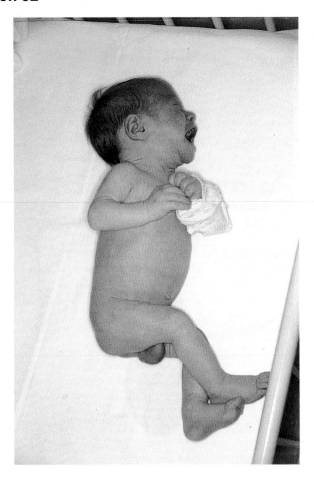

An infant of 3 months was admitted with a left lower lobe pneumonia. Electrolyte analysis revealed a hyponatraemic metabolic alkalosis. There was failure to thrive with a weight below the third centile.

a) What features are shown above?
b) What is the likely diagnosis? Explain the electrolyte result.

Answer to Question 52

a) Abdominal distension
   Paucity of subcutaneous fat
b) Cystic fibrosis (CF)
   Pseudo Bartter syndrome

- CF is a well-recognized cause of failure to thrive.
- Presentation of CF includes: failure to thrive (45%); recurrent respiratory symptoms (40%); meconium ileus (10%) and others such as obstructive neonatal jaundice, anaemia with oedema, heat exhaustion, rectal prolapse and via screening.
- Neonatal screening: serum immunoreactive trypsin levels (IRT) confirmed by sweat testing at 3–4 weeks of age. The IRT is unreliable in neonates after surgery for meconium ileus.
- Equivocal sweat tests may be differentiated by the fludrocortisone suppression test which suppresses electrolyte levels in most normals. Increased electrical potentials across the nasal mucosa are used in difficult cases.
- Pseudo Bartter syndrome occurs due to electrolyte loss and is characterized by hyponatraemia, hypokalaemia and a metabolic alkalosis.
- The most common gene deletion has been determined on chromosome 7q (68% in N W Europe). The gene product, CF trans-membrane regulator, lacks a phenylalanine residue at position 508, accounting for changes in chloride ion permeability in CF.

David T J 1990 Cystic fibrosis. Arch. Dis. Child. 65:152–157
Tizzano E F, Buchwald M 1992 Cystic fibrosis: beyond the gene to therapy. J. Pediatr. 120:337–349

Question 53

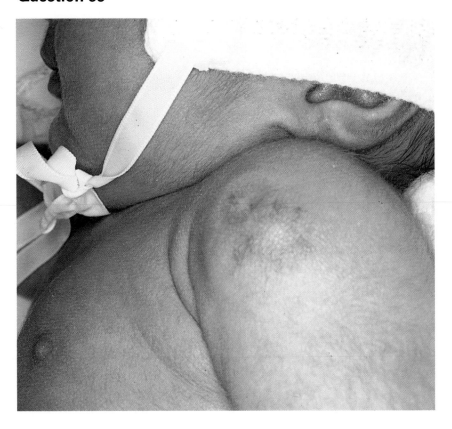

This Asian infant presented at 6 weeks of age with the above abnormality. Examination revealed palpable axillary lymph nodes.

a) What is the diagnosis?
b) Give two other complications.

Answer to Question 53

a) Incorrect BCG vaccination causing an abscess
b) Ulceration
Keloid formation
Suppurative lymphadenitis
Anaphylaxis
Dissemination of organisms
Lupoid type of local lesion

- BCG vaccination was first introduced in 1921.
- Protection rates are quoted up to 80%. About 90% of vaccines are tuberculin positive at 4–5 years of age after neonatal vaccination.
- Neonatal vaccination seems to offer better protection against tuberculous meningitis and other disseminated forms than pulmonary disease.
- Administration must be intradermal. Subcutaneous injection may be responsible for ulcers and abscess formation. Lymphadenitis is common.
- Groups for whom neonatal vaccination is advised are: Asian babies or those of other immigrant families with a high infection rate; infants travelling in high risk areas; those in contact with active respiratory disease and those born into families with a history of TB within the last 5 years. HIV testing prior to neonatal vaccination is not required.

Clarke A, Rudd P 1992 Neonatal BCG immunisation. Arch. Dis. Child. 67:473–474

Question 54

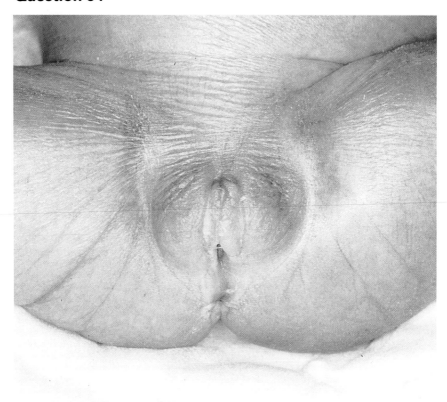

This newborn infant has a cleft palate, abnormal hands and the dermatological problem illustrated.

a) What is the connection between these abnormalities?
b) What urgent investigation is required?
c) Comment upon the likely growth and development of this child.

Answer to Question 54

a) EEC syndrome: ectodermal dysplasia
                    ectrodactyly
                    cleft palate.
b) Renal ultrasound to detect urinary tract abnormalities commonly associated with the syndrome, particularly renal agenesis, hydronephrosis and ureteric duplication.
c) Normal growth and life span. Some individuals may have psychomotor delay.

- First reported in 1970. Autosomal dominant with variable penetrance although sporadic cases occur. No gender preference.
- Ectrodactyly is invariable affecting hands and feet. The third digit may be absent or dysplastic.
- Ectodermal dysplasia may be associated with atresia of the nasolacrimal duct. Hair is fine and sparse whilst teeth and nails may be hypoplastic. Hyperkeratosis may occur.
- Urinary tract defects are common.
- Other problems include: increased susceptibility to eye infections due to persistent tearing; dental caries resulting from reduced salivation and, rarely, microcephaly.
- Asymptomatic carriers may be detected by hand radiographs or by detection of minimal palatal clefts or velopharyngeal insufficiency.

Question 55

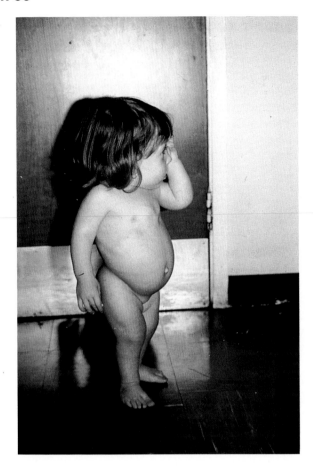

a) Give three possible causes for this child's short stature.
b) Give two useful investigations to aid diagnosis.
c) What possible new therapeutic modalities may be of benefit to such children?

Answer to Question 55

a) Skeletal dysplasia–spondylo-epimetaphyseal dysplasia congenita in this case
Mucopolysaccharidosis
Atypical achondroplasia
Dwarfism syndromes
b) Skeletal survey
Bone age (less use when there is an abnormal skeleton)
Urinalysis for mucopolysaccharides
c) Recombinant growth hormone (wider therapeutic indication on trial only)
Surgical limb lengthening

- Spondylo-epimetaphyseal dysplasia congenita is characterized by:
  short limbed dwarfism from birth
    mild facial dysmorphism with high palate and hypertelorism
  kyphoscoliosis
    pectus carinatum and, latterly, hip contractures.
- Ossification is retarded and seen in the spine, proximal femur and pubis. C2 vertebrae may be hypoplastic.
- Autosomal dominant with equal sex predominance. Incidence is 1:100 000.
- Genetic abnormality is mapped to chromosome 12q. Molecular defect may be excessive post-translational modification of collagen.
- Complications include: hypotonia, myopia, retinal detachment, hearing loss and cataracts.

Question 56

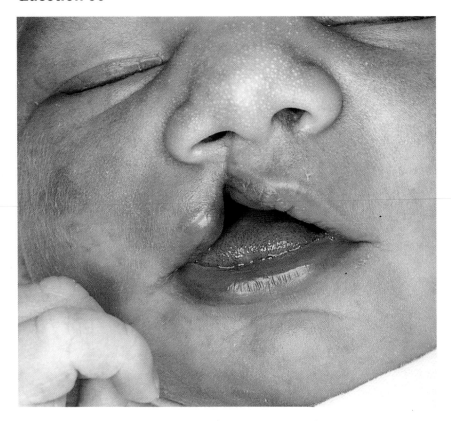

This infant has a cleft lip associated with a cleft palate.

a) List four problems which may be encountered in the care of this child.
b) Give four syndromes associated with cleft lip or palate.

Answer to Question 56

a) Feeding difficulties–poor sucking and regurgitation
Recurrent otitis media with subsequent chronic serous otitis
Speech delay
Abnormal development of dentition
Hearing loss due to serous otitis
Cosmetic concerns
Difficult parental bonding and psychological problems when older
b) Pierre–Robin syndrome
Trisomy 13
Fetal phenytoin syndrome
Goldenhar syndrome
Orofacial digital syndrome
EEC syndrome

- Many units perform early neonatal cleft lip repair. This is still debated. Palatal surgery is performed within the first year.
- Most common presentation is unilateral (left side) cleft.
- Cleft lip +/− palate occurs in 1:1000 live births with a sex ratio of 2:1 male:female. The risk of recurrence is 1:25 if there is no parental occurrence or 1:10 if a parent is affected.
- The aetiology is multifactorial.
- Adenoidectomy should be avoided if possible as removal may increase the nasality of speech and food regurgitation.

Question 57

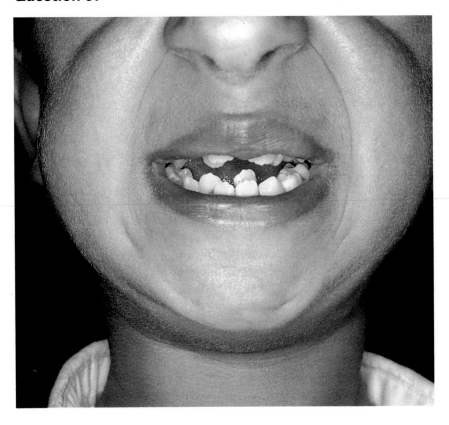

This Asian boy presented with short stature.

a) What is the most likely diagnosis?
b) What is the possible mode of inheritance?

Answer to Question 57

a) Pyknodysostosis
b) Autosomal recessive

- Pyknodysostosis is characterized by:
  Short stature
  Increased tendency to fracture
  Delayed closure of sutures
  Facial and palatal hypoplasia
  Irregular and delayed dentition
  Atrophic terminal phalanges.
- X-rays show generalized osteosclerosis.
- Although similar to Albers–Schönberg disease, cranial nerve entrapment and haematological complications do not occur.

Barr D G D 1992 Diseases of bone. In: Campbell A G M, McIntosh N (eds). Forfar and Arneil's textbook of paediatrics, 4th edn. Churchill Livingstone, Edinburgh

Question 58

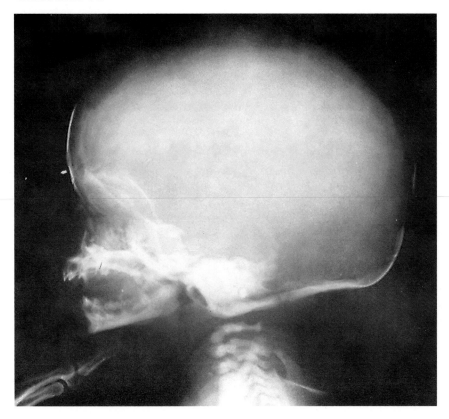

a) What does this neonatal skull radiograph show?
b) What is the risk of recurrence to future siblings?

Answer to Question 58

a) Occipital encephalocele
b) Approximately 5%

- Encephaloceles are often midline and predominantly occipital. They arise following failure of normal development of the neural tube.
- Large encephaloceles are associated with severe neurological dysfunction and hydrocephalus.
- Treatment is neurosurgical.
- Incidence is 1:2000 live births.
- Differentiation from haemangiomata and scalp tumours is necessary. Encephaloceles are rarely covered in hair. Ultrasound may be of help.

Madden N P, Cudmore R E 1991 Scalp tumours mimicking encephaloceles. Arch. Dis. Child. 66:884–885

Question 59

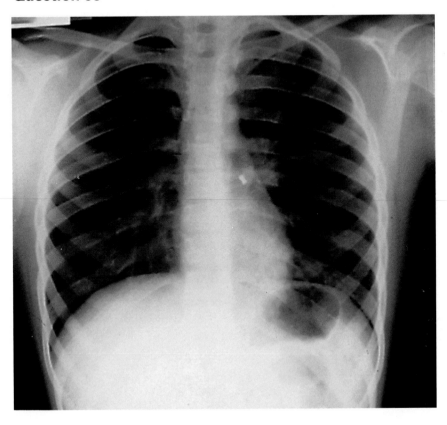

A 13-year-old girl presented with an episode of coughing and wheezing. Auscultation revealed reduced breath sounds and some crepitations in the left lower zone. This is her chest X-ray.

a) What other investigation is indicated in this case? Why?

Answer to Question 59

a) Lateral chest X-ray.

The PA chest X-ray suggests the presence of a foreign body in the left bronchial system. The physical signs could be consistent with the aspiration of a foreign body. However, it is unusual for a teenager to aspirate a radio-opaque foreign body and its position is also unusual as the right bronchial system is more commonly affected. A lateral chest X-ray is shown below:

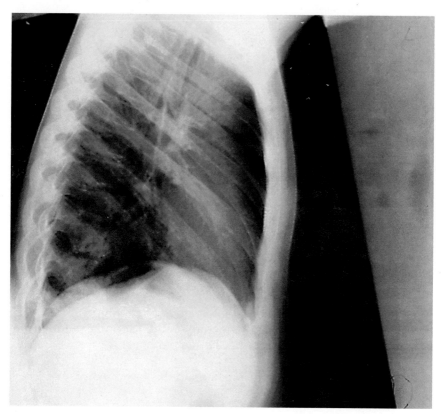

The lateral film shows that the foreign body is not intrathoracic but is part of a hair clip seen in the top left of the X-ray! It also demonstrates the left lower lobe pneumonia responsible for the clinical signs. A classic trap for the unwary!

Question 60

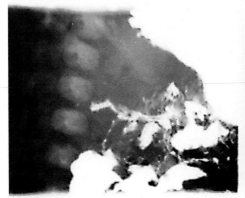 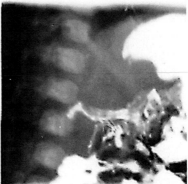

A 4-week-old girl was admitted with a 2 week history of persistent vomiting.

a) What radiological procedure has been performed? Diagnosis?

b) List three other useful investigations. Outline your management of this case.

Answer to Question 60

a) Barium meal
   Hypertrophic pyloric stenosis—elongation and partial narrowing of
   the pyloric canal is shown
b) Test feed to demonstrate visible peristalsis and palpable pyloric
   tumour
   Pyloric ultrasound
   Electrolyte and acid-base analysis
   Urinary pH estimation

   Cessation of feeding
   Correction of dehydration, electrolyte imbalance and metabolic
   alkalosis
   Surgical pyloromyotomy
   Early postoperative feeding

- Commonly affects firstborn males. Male:female ratio 4:1. Incidence
  3:1000 live births.
- Vomiting usually starts at 2–3 weeks of age but may date from birth.
  Projectile vomiting is not invariable.
- Vomitus never contains bile. Blood is detected in 20% of cases.
- Pyloric ultrasound is suggestive of stenosis when the measured
  muscle thickness exceeds 4 mm. Barium meal may reveal the
  'string' sign due to the compression of the barium through a
  narrowed canal.
- Classic electrolyte imbalance shows a hypokalaemic, hypochlor-
  aemic metabolic alkalosis with a paradoxical acidic urinary pH.
- Persistent postoperative vomiting may be due to an incomplete
  procedure, gastro-oesophageal reflux (more common with pyloric
  stenosis cases than the general population) or sepsis (UTI).

Question 61

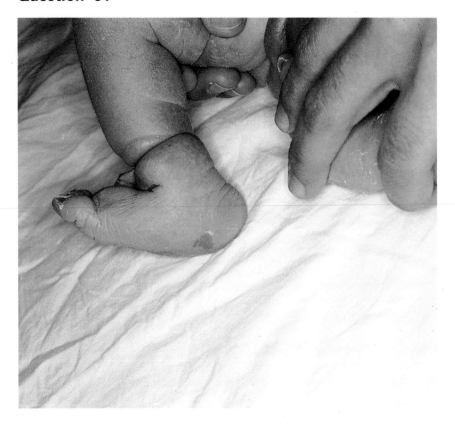

a) What is the diagnosis?

Answer to Question 61

a) Disruption due to a constriction ring resulting from an amniotic band.

- Incidence unknown but uncommon.
- Aetiology unknown: a widely accepted theory is that a first trimester amnion rupture, followed by herniation of the fetus into a false cavity between the chorion and amnion, allows the membranes to encircle and constrict the fetus. Another theory postulates a vascular accident.
- Craniofacial abnormalities may co-exist.

Question 62

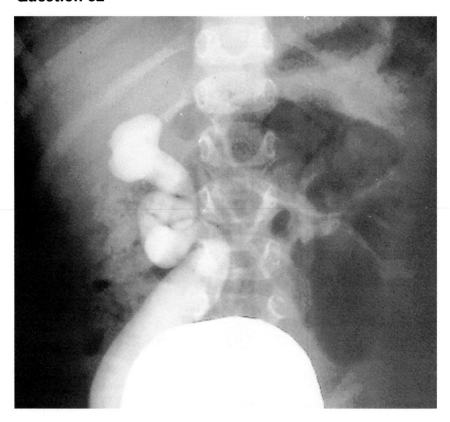

A child was investigated following a urinary tract infection.

a) What investigation has been performed?
b) Describe the findings of this test.
c) Give another useful investigation to aid your management.

Answer to Question 62

a) Intravenous urogram (IVU)
b) Distended bladder
   Right hydro-ureter
   Right renal clubbed calyces
   These findings are consistent with severe right vesico-ureteric reflux
c) DMSA renal scan to detect renal scarring
   DTPA renal scan to assess renal function

- Urinary tract infection (UTI) is common: 3–5% of girls; 0.5–2% of boys.
- Vesico-ureteric reflux (VUR) occurs in 30% of those with UTI.
- VUR resolves in 80% by mid childhood. 30% with VUR sustain renal scarring, usually in the first infection.
- 10–20% of those with VUR and renal scarring develop hypertension. VUR is the commonest cause of paediatric end stage renal failure.
- Obstructive lesions are detected in 7% of children with UTI.
- All children with UTI require investigation. The nature of this depends upon the age of the child:

<1 year:
1. Renal ultrasound during acute episode.
2. Plain abdominal X-ray to detect calculi and spinal defects.
3. Micturating cysto-urethrogram (MCUG) when the urine is sterile to exclude reflux.
4. DMSA scan (more sensitive than ultrasound at detecting renal scars although if performed too soon after the UTI, areas of renal hypoperfusion may incorrectly mimic scars).

1–7 years:
1. Renal ultrasound.
2. Abdominal X-ray.
3. DMSA scan (IVU if DMSA is not available).
4. DTPA or MCUG only in recurrent sepsis /+ve family history for VUR.

Working Group 1991: Guidelines for the management of acute UTI in childhood. J. Roy. Coll. Phy. Lond. 25(1):36–41

Question 63

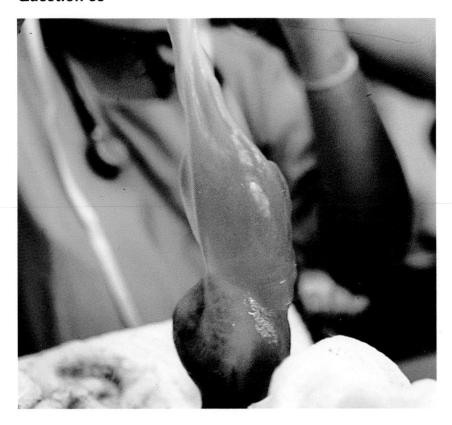

a) What is the abnormality shown?
b) What other condition must be differentiated from this?

Answer to Question 63

a) Omphalocele (exomphalos)
b) Gastroschisis–there is no sac covering the defect and the umbilical cord is inserted at the edge of the defect

- Incidence of 1:10 000 live births.
- Up to 50% have associated cardiovascular, genito-urinary or GI abnormalities.
- Management includes: reducing evaporational losses by occlusive film; free drainage of gastric secretions; adequate hydration with i.v. fluids; plasma for hypotension; measurement of renal output and assessment/treatment of associated defects. Surgical repair.
- Complications include: respiratory embarrassment due to raised intra-abdominal pressure after repair; IVC obstruction; renal vein thrombosis; gut ischaemia and sepsis.

Question 64

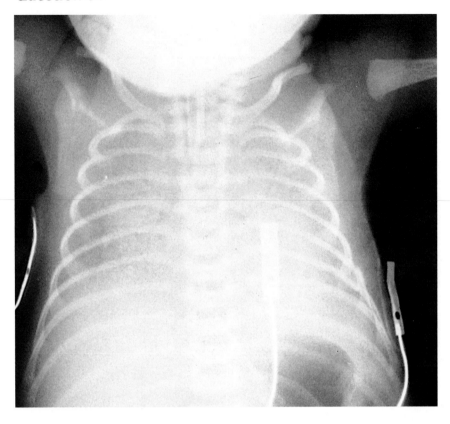

A neonate developed respiratory signs shortly after birth resulting in mechanical ventilation. There was a history of prolonged rupture of maternal membranes and pyrexia. This is the chest X-ray.

a) Give two possible diagnoses.
b) Despite adequate ventilation, this child remained hypoxic. Why? How would you correct this?

Answer to Question 64

a) Neonatal sepsis–Group B haemolytic streptococci (GBHS) in this
case
Hyaline membrane disease–can occur in term babies
b) Pulmonary hypertension (persistent fetal circulation) due to sepsis
Cyanotic cardiac disease needs to be excluded
Increasing oxygenation by: tolazoline infusion
prostacyclin infusion
magnesium sulphate
ECMO (extracorporeal membrane
oxygenation)

- 15% of pregnant women may be colonized with GBHS. 1% of
  colonized infants develop invasive disease.
- Mortality is high (20–30%). Early disease is septicaemic but meningitis often co-exists. Neurodevelopmental handicap may reach 50%
  of survivors.
- Presenting features and radiographic changes may be identical to
  those of hyaline membrane disease.
- Pulmonary hypertension and hypoxaemia often occur due to
  cytokine and free radical release. Pulmonary hypertension is
  partially mediated by thromboxane. Prostacyclin is of benefit by
  antagonizing thromboxane, causing vasodilatation and preventing
  platelet aggregation.
- ECMO is often used in the USA. Quoted survival rates are in excess
  of 77%.

Abu-Osba Y K 1991 Treatment of persistent pulmonary hypertension of
the newborn: an update. Arch. Dis. Child. 66:74–77
Brutocao D P, O'Rourke P P 1992 Extracorporeal membrane oxygenation. In: David T J (ed) Recent advances in paediatrics. Churchill
Livingstone, Edinburgh

Question 65

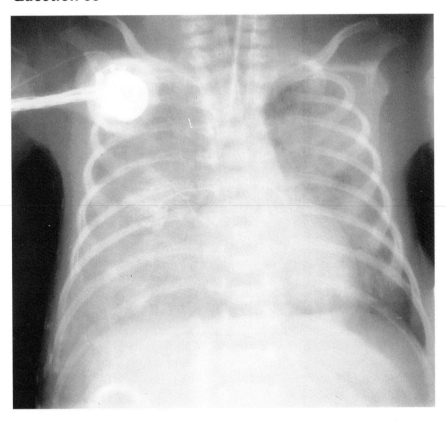

A preterm infant of 27 weeks' gestation, ventilated for hyaline membrane disease, collapsed with hypotension and hypoxia. The baby was receiving antibiotics and parenteral nutrition through a percutaneous silastic long line inserted via a right antecubital vein. This is the chest X-ray after dye has been injected down the catheter.

a) What is the diagnosis?
b) How may this have occurred?

Answer to Question 65

a) Right pleural collection (of TPN in this case) and pneumonitis.

b) Incorrect catheter position, either as a result of incorrect placement or catheter migration, in the pulmonary vasculature causes over-load and rupture of the capillary system. TPN may therefore leak into the interstitium, then into the alveoli or the pleural space.

Management is by pleural tap; bronchial lavage; antibiotics; increased ventilation; removal of the catheter and possibly steroids.

- The ideal position for such a catheter is with the tip lying at the right atrium.
- Other catheter associated complications include:
Sepsis–often coagulase negative staphylococci (3–15%)
Blockage
Thrombophlebitis
Thrombosis
Malpositioning leading to pulmonary complications and to subdural effusions if inserted into tributaries of the SVC.

Rubin S, Hewson P, Roberton N R C 1986 Pulmonary complications of total parenteral nutrition in a neonate. J. Roy. Soc. Med. 79:545–547
Young S, MacMahon P, Kovar I Z 1989 Subdural intravenous fat collection: an unusual complication of central intravenous feeding in the neonate. J. Parentr. Enter. Nutr. 13:661

Question 66

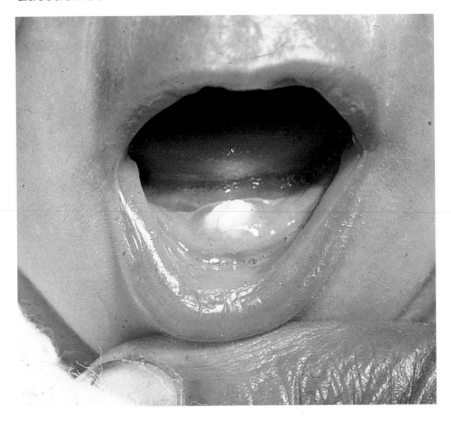

a) What is the diagnosis?
b) What are the common associations?
c) What is the appropriate action?

Answer to Question 66

a) Congenital tooth.

b) Usually an isolated finding; described associations are of cleft palate, Pierre–Robin syndrome, Ellis van Creveld syndrome and others.

c) Tooth extraction is undertaken because of the risk of detachment and subsequent aspiration, and the maternal discomfort during breast feeding.

- Incidence approximately 1:2000 newborns.
- Usually they are mandibular central incisors.
- Attachment of congenital teeth is generally limited to the gingival margin, with little root formation or body support, hence their removal is easy.
- It might be a prematurely erupted primary tooth, in which case early eruption may be expected.
- There is a family history of congenital teeth or premature eruption in 15–20% of affected children.

Question 67

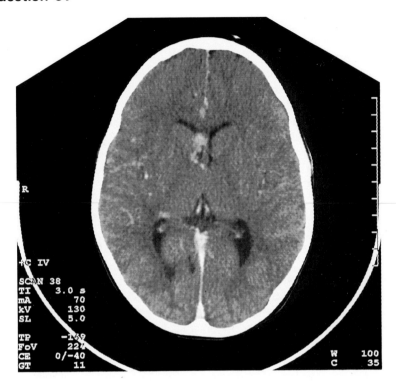

A 3-year-old boy was admitted following a prolonged seizure. This CT brain scan was performed.

a) Describe the radiological abnormality.
b) What is the diagnosis?
c) List three other features of your diagnosis.

Answer to Question 67

a) Several areas of nodular intracranial calcification next to the ventricular system
b) Tuberous sclerosis (TS)
c) Facial angiofibromas ('adenoma sebaceum')
Periungual fibromas
Calcified retinal hamartomas
Multiple cortical tubers
Bilateral renal angiomyolipomas
Others include: shagreen patch; fibrous forehead patch; cardiac rhabdomyomas; hypomelanotic macules; pulmonary lymphangioleiomyomatosis (honeycomb lung)

- Autosomal dominant inheritance — 70% arise as a new mutation.
- All seizure types may occur in TS.
- 65% of seizures at onset are of infantile spasm type.
- Age of seizure and degree of mental handicap are related.
- Hypomelanotic macules are often best seen with a Wood's light.
- Over 50% of children will develop rhabdomyomas.
- Cranial CT may be normal in the first year of life.
- Abnormal gene location on 9q and 11q.

Webb DW, Osborne JP 1992 Tuberous sclerosis. In: David TJ (ed) Recent Advances in Paediatrics, Vol 11. Churchill Livingstone, Edinburgh, pp. 147-160

Question 68

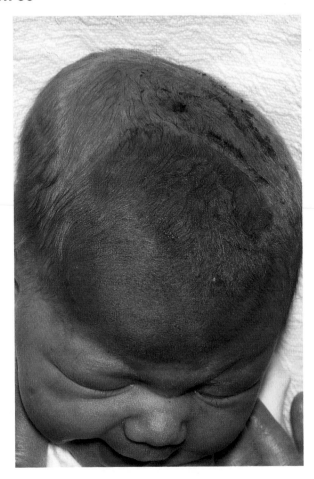

a) What is the diagnosis?
b) What obstetric procedure was performed?
c) What is the natural history?

Answer to Question 68

a) Right parietal cephalhaematoma and vacuum chignon

b) Vacuum extraction

c) Most cephalhaematomas are resorbed within 2 weeks to 3 months, depending on their size. A few remain as bony protuberances for years, after being calcified, and are detectable on skull X-ray as widening of the diploic tissue.

- Cephalhaematomas are usually not visible until several hours after birth, since subperiosteal bleeding is a slow process.
- An underlying skull fracture, usually linear and not depressed, is occasionally associated with cephalhaematomas.
- Cephalhaematomas may begin to calcify by the end of the second week.

Question 69

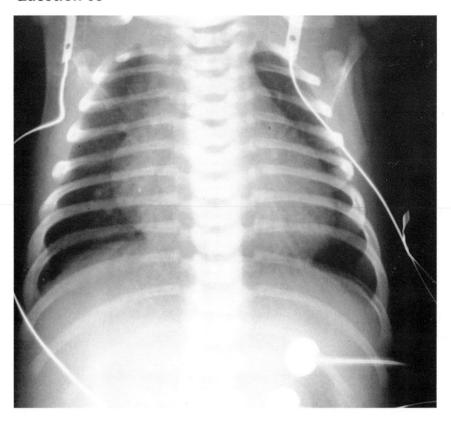

This is a chest X-ray of a 2-day-old neonate, who presented with cardiovascular collapse and acidaemia.

a) What is the likely diagnosis?
b) What urgent investigations would you undertake?
c) What urgent therapeutic intervention is needed?

Answer to Question 69

a) Left ventricular outflow tract (LVOT) obstruction, although the possibility of overwhelming sepsis should be covered.

b) Assessment of the 4 limb pulses and blood pressure
ECG
Cross-sectional echocardiogram (when available)
Infection screen

c) Prostaglandin infusion
Mechanical ventilation
Broad spectrum antibiotics
Referral to a cardiac centre

- The neonate who presents with heart failure and refractory acidosis during the first or second week of life is a paediatric emergency; left-sided obstructive lesions with duct dependent circulation account for the majority of cases.
- Absence of the femoral pulses is diagnostic of coarctation of the aorta.
- Absence of one pulse (left arm = interuption of aortic arch) or generally poor pulses (aortic atresia, left hypoplastic ventricle syndrome, congenital cardiomyopathy) may give further clues to the diagnosis.
- The major differential diagnosis in the severely acidotic collapsed infant is overwhelming sepsis.
- Obstructed total anomalous pulmonary venous return (TAPVR) may also present similarly, when the ductus venosus closes; a CXR, though, would show pulmonary oedema *without cardiomegaly.*

Redington A N 1991 Clinical assessment of the neonate and infant with suspected congenital heart disease: how to avoid some of the pitfalls. Curr. Paediatr. 1:65–72

Question 70

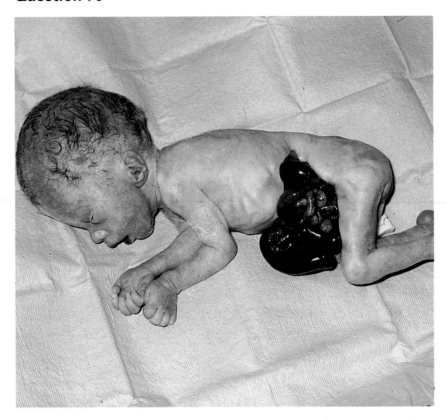

a) What is the diagnosis?
b) What immediate actions would you take after birth?
c) What other major abnormalities are associated with this condition?

Answer to Question 70

a) Gastroschisis

b) Prevent heat and fluid loss, by covering the defect
   Correct hypoproteinaemia, by giving sufficient plasma
   Prevent abdominal distention, by passing a large nasogastric tube
   Refer for surgery

c) Intestinal atresia

- Incidence of 1:6000 is increasing in recent years.
- Lethal abnormalities are rare (unlike exomphalos). Frequent association is intra-uterine growth retardation.
- Extensive protein losses occur into the bowel and peritoneal cavity.
- Surgical replacement of the intestine in the peritoneal cavity in one or two stage procedure is performed. Bowel resection for ischaemic damage is sometimes required.
- Intravenous nutrition occasionally is required for weeks or months.
- The mode of delivery does not affect the outcome but optimal postnatal care is essential.

Stringer M D, Brereton R J, Wright V M 1991 Controversies in the management of gastroschisis: a study of 40 patients. Arch. Dis. Child. 66:34–36

Question 71

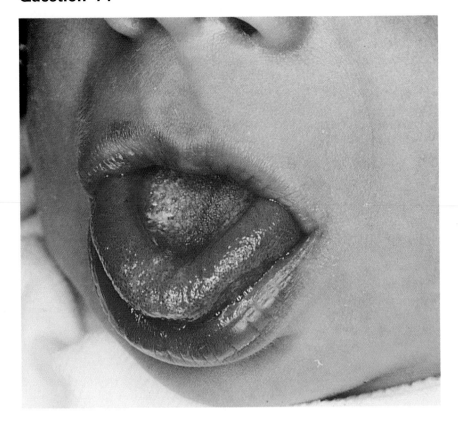

This neonate underwent surgical repair for exomphalos minor soon after birth.

a) What is the diagnosis?
b) What immediate investigation would you perform soon after birth?
c) Give one investigation that should be performed for the first 3 to 5 years of life.

Answer to Question 71

a) Beckwith–Wiedemann syndrome
b) Blood glucose to exclude hypoglycaemia
c) Serial abdominal ultrasound scans for neoplasia

- Incidence of 1:14 000 births.
- Beckwith is a professor in paediatric pathology at Washington University with interest in tumour pathogenesis and classification of Wilms tumour.
- The clinical features of B–W syndrome are:
  Anterior abdominal wall defect (90%)
  High birth weight
  Macroglossia (90%)
  Ear lobe grooves
  Hemihypertrophy (15%).
- Neonatal hypoglycaemia due to hyperinsulinaemia may occur (30–50%) and result in mental retardation if untreated.
- Neoplasias, especially Wilms tumour or adrenal cortical carcinoma, occur in 7.5% (40% if hemihypertophy is present, 3% if absent) and merit 3-monthly abdominal ultrasound scans for the first years of life.
- B–W syndrome may be aetiologically heterogeneous, as a small duplication of chromosome 11p15 has been found in some patients; those with the 11p15 duplication are more prone to neoplasias. It is interesting that the same duplication is found in infants with neoplasias (i.e. Wilms tumour), but no features of B–W syndrome.

Connor J M, Ferguson–Smith M A 1987 Congenital malformations. In: Connor J M, Ferguson–Smith M A (eds) Essential medical genetics. Blackwell, Oxford

Question 72

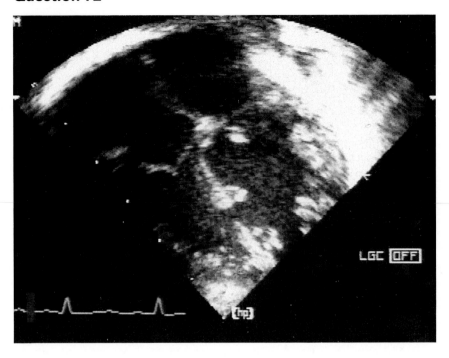

This is a cross-sectional echocardiogram (4 chamber view) of a newborn.

a) What is the abnormality?
b) What is the prognosis?
c) How would you manage this patient?

Answer to Question 72

a) Ventricular septal defect–VSD (echogenic drop out half way through the 'thick' ventricular septum).

b) The prognosis depends on the size and the position of the VSD and the physiological changes, which take place as a result of blood flowing through the defect. Small defects usually close spontaneously, most of them during the first 1–2 years of life. Large defects may lead to congestive heart failure, with a potential for pulmonary hypertension.

c) Exclude other associated cardiac abnormalities
Early follow-up (4–6 weeks)
Medical treatment for heart failure
Surgical closure if heart failure is poorly controlled or signs of pulmonary hypertension develop
Provide SBE prophylaxis, when indicated.

- The pulmonary vascular resistance in healthy newborns decreases by 7–10 days; in patients with a VSD this is delayed to 4–6 weeks, hence the fact the large VSDs often are not clinically detectable during the first month of life.
- The early recognition of developing pulmonary vascular disease is based on the assessment of the pulmonary component of the second heart sound (loud P2).
- The doubly committed subarterial defects have a potential for acquired infundibular pulmonary stenosis and tetralogy of Fallot physiology.
- Aortic regurgitation may complicate subaortic VSD later on in childhood as a result of prolapse of the coronary cusps, predominantly right, into the VSD.

Anderson R H, Shinebourne E A et al 1987 Ventricular septal defect. In: Anderson R H, Shinebourne E A (eds) Paediatric cardiology. Churchill Livingstone, Edinburgh

Question 73

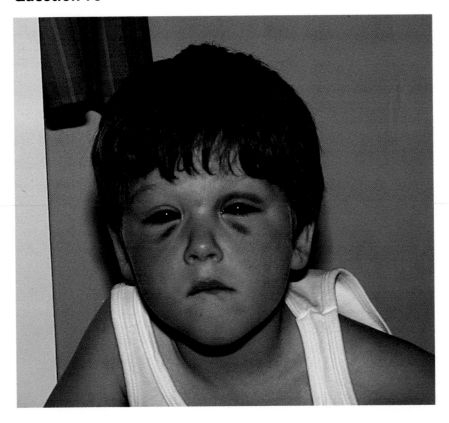

This toddler presented to his GP with a history of paroxysmal cough following coryzal symptoms.

a) What is the diagnosis?
b) What is the aetiological factor?
c) What is the treatment?

Answer to Question 73

a) Pertussis

b) *Bordetella pertussis.* Identical clinical picture can be due to *Bordetella parapertussis, Bordetella bronchiseptica,* adenoviruses, parainfluenza and RSV.

c) Supportive treatment: maintenance of hydration and nutrition and oxygen with nasopharyngeal suction when needed.

- Pertussis has been described as the '100 day cough'.
- Pneumonia, usually due to secondary bacterial invaders, is responsible for more than 90% of deaths under the age of 3.
- An inspiratory whoop is not always seen in infants and older children or adults.
- Subconjuctival haemorrhages are common; during coughing paroxysms the intrathoracic pressure rises sharply and affects the venous return to the heart. The sudden surges in capillary pressure may rupture the poorly supported subconjuctival vessels and produce alarming haemorrhages.
- *Bordetella pertussis* can be isolated from as many as 90% of patients during the catarrhal stage of the disease, but from less than 50% during the paroxysmal stage.

Question 74

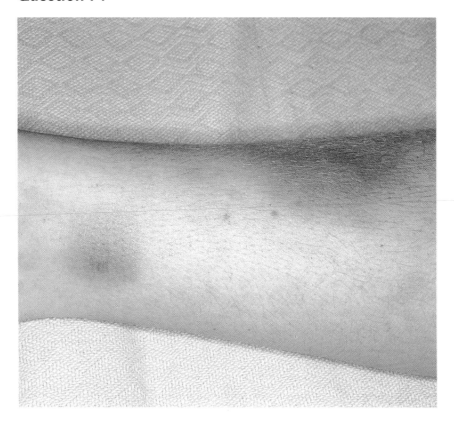

This child presented with spontaneous bruising and a platelet count of 10. She was otherwise well without hepatosplenomegaly or lymphadenopathy.

a) What is the likely diagnosis?
b) How do you confirm this?
c) What is your acute management?

Answer to Question 74

a) Idiopathic thrombocytopenic purpura (ITP)
b) By excluding other causes of thrombocytopenia (e.g. leukaemias). If the diagnosis is in doubt bone marrow examination is mandatory.
c) Admit to hospital to establish the diagnosis
   Reassure the family about the benign nature of the condition
   Reserve steroids or intravenous immunoglobulin for overt bleeding.

- Hepatosplenomegaly or lymphadenopathy are not features of ITP and suggest another diagnosis.
- Bone marrow examination is mandatory in all cases of presumed ITP if steroids are to be given.
- 90% of acute ITP remits spontaneously within 3 months and the rest within 6 months; persistence longer than 6 months is considered chronic.
- Mortality of childhood ITP is less than 1%.
- Whilst splenectomy is effective in raising platelets, it is rarely indicated in view of the risk of post-splenectomy fatal sepsis. This risk has been estimated at 1.4% compared to less than 1% mortality rate from ITP.
- Intravenous immunoglobulin is the treatment of choice post-trauma or pre-operatively.
- In the event of intracranial haemorrhage the following should be urgently performed:
  Massive allogenic platelet transfusion
  High dose intravenous immunoglobulin infusion
  Emergency splenectomy.
  The above measures reduce the mortality rate to 50%.

Eden O B, Lilleyman J S 1992 Guidelines for management of idiopathic thrombocytopenic purpura. Arch. Dis. Child. 67:1056–1058
Lilleyman J S 1990 Changing perspectives in idiopathic thrombocytopenic purpura. In: Meadow R (ed) Recent advances in paediatrics, Vol 8. Churchill Livingstone, Edinburgh

Question 75

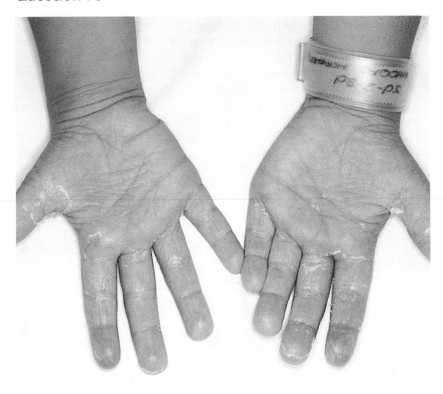

These are the hands of a toddler who is recovering from a 14 day acute febrile illness associated with conjunctivitis, pharyngitis and a generalized erythematous rash.

a) What is the likely diagnosis?
b) What important investigation should be undertaken as soon as the diagnosis is made or suspected?
c) What is the treatment?

Answer to Question 75

a) Kawasaki disease or mucocutaneous lymph node syndrome.
b) Cross-sectional echocardiography for detection of coronary artery lesions.
c) Aspirin is given in the acute phase and then in a reduced antiplatelet dose in the presence of coronary artery involvement.
Gammaglobulin intravenously, during the acute phase of the disease.

- Kawasaki disease is an immunologically mediated diffuse vasculitis of childhood of unknown aetiology.
- The diagnosis is made when five of the six following criteria are satisfied:
Fever longer than 5 days
Conjunctival injection
Mucous membrane changes: erythema, fissuring and crusting of the lips, strawberry tongue
Erythematous rash
Lymphadenopathy
Changes in the extremities (late onset): induration of hand and feet, erythema of palms and toes, desquamation of finger and toe tips.
- A neutrophil leucocytosis, thrombocytosis and a high ESR are commonly seen, but no organisms have been cultured and auto-antibodies are negative.
- Cardiac involvement, ranging from pericardial effusion to coronary artery aneurysm is the most important manifestation of the disease.
- 10 to 40% of cases will have echocardiographic evidence of coronary vasculitis within 2 weeks of the illness.
- Coronary involvement is significantly associated with leucocytosis and thrombocytosis.
- Most coronary lesions regress; good prognostic factors are: age less than 1 year, female sex, fusiform aneurysm and maximum diameter less than 4 mm.
- Currently intravenous gammaglobulin is given routinely on diagnosis (single dose of 2 g/kg i.v. over 10–12hrs); when given early in the disease prevents cardiac involvement and even late administration provides some symptomatic relief.

Barron K S 1991 Kawasaki disease. Epidemiology, late prognosis and therapy. Rheum. Dis. Clin. N. Amer. 17(4):907–919
Tizard E J, Suzuki A, Levin M, Dillon M J 1991 Clinical aspects of 100 patients with Kawasaki disease. Arch. Dis. Child. 66:185–188

Question 76

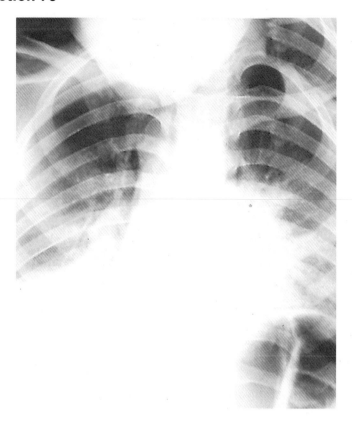

This is a chest X-ray of a 12-year-old boy, presenting with a 1 week history of pyrexia and cough and minimal respiratory signs on examination.

a) What is the likely diagnosis?
b) What laboratory tests are indicated?
c) How would you treat this condition?

Answer to Question 76

a) Mycoplasma pneumonia.
b) Cold agglutinins
Throat/sputum culture
Acute/convalescent serology
Blood cultures for other organisms.
c) Full therapeutic dose of erythromycin or tetracyclines (children over the age of 8) for approximately 7 days after defervescence; they both ameliorate the clinical course but do not eradicate the organism.

- Mycoplasma infections are common amongst older children and young adults.
- Only 3–10% of cases present as pneumonia; the rest of them usually present as URTIs, tracheobronchitis, etc.
- Cold agglutinins, which are specific haemagglutinins reacting to the I antigen of red blood cells, are usually the first antibodies detected; they are present in 33–67% of cases, usually during the second week, disappearing in about 6 weeks. Their presence and their titres correlate well with the severity of the illness.
- A new DNA probe assay on sputum as a rapid diagnostic testing is now becoming available.
- White cell count is normal.
- Complications are rashes, erythema multiforme, meningo-encephalitis, transverse myelitis and Guillain–Barré syndrome. Mild degrees of haemolysis 2–3 weeks after the onset of illness is common; severe haemolysis, thrombocytopenia and coagulation defects are uncommon. Finally myocarditis, pericarditis and rheumatic fever-like syndrome have been reported.
- Previous infections as demonstrated by the presence of circulating antibodies do not seem to confer lifelong immunity on children.
- *Mycoplasma pneumoniae* is the most common infectious cause of acute chest syndrome in sickle cell patients.

Kleemola S R, Karjalainen J E, Riaty R K 1990 Rapid diagnosis of *Mycoplasma pneumoniae* infection: clinical evaluation of a commercial probe test. J. Infect. Dis. 162:70–75
Nagayama Y, Sakurai N et al 1988 Isolation of *Mycoplasma pneumoniae* from children with lower respiratory tract infections. J. Infect. Dis. 157:911–917

Question 77

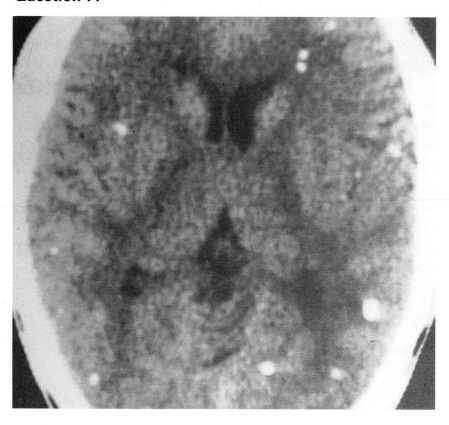

This is a cranial CT of a neonate who presented with hepatospleno-megaly and convulsions.

a) What is the likely diagnosis?
b) How do you confirm the diagnosis?
c) What single investigation can be an aid to diagnosis and needs to be repeated during early childhood?

Answer to Question 77

a) Congenital toxoplasmosis (CMV infection calcifications are peri-ventricular).
b) By specific serology; absence of toxoplasma specific IgM in the neonatal serum does not exclude the diagnosis as 50% of infected newborns do not mount IgM response; persistence of the toxo-plasmosis IgG by the age of 1 year confirms the diagnosis.
Alternatively whole neonatal blood can be tested for the presence of toxoplasma DNA using a polymerase chain reaction.
c) Ophthalmoscopy; chorioretinitis develops in the majority of cases (up to 90%) even as late as 20 years.

- Only 10–15% of congenitally infected infants are symptomatic at birth; the 'classic triad' of chorioretinitis, intracranial calcifications and hydrocephalus is seen in only 3%.
- The risk of vertical transmission in untreated mothers is approxi-mately 25% during the first trimester, increasing to 65% when the infection develops in the last trimester. Conversely the risk for severe disease in the fetus is higher when transmission occurs early in pregnancy.
- The value of antenatal treatment with spiramicin (plus pyrime-thamine and a sulphonamide, when the fetus is infected) is well established; it reduces the vertical transmission rate and also the severity of disease in the newborn.
- Pregnant women should avoid cat litter, wash fruit and vegetables thoroughly and should only eat well cooked meat to prevent gestational toxoplasmosis.
- The fetus is not at risk of congenital toxoplasmosis if the mother has seroconverted in the past.

Hall S M 1992 Congenital toxoplasmosis. Br. Med. J. 305:291–297
Remington J S, Desmonts G 1990 Toxoplasmosis. In: Remington J S, Klein J Q (eds) Infectious diseases of the fetus and newborn infant. W B Saunders, Philadelphia

Question 78

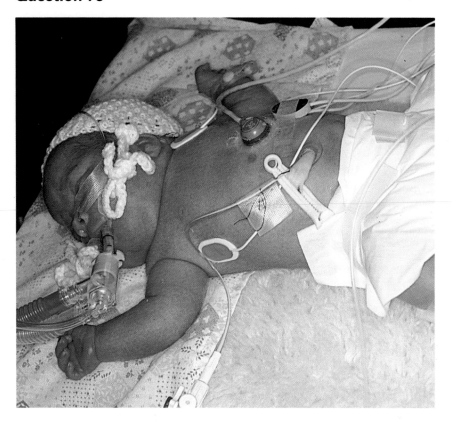

This infant was born at 33 weeks' gestation to a diabetic mother.

a) How could you predict the likelihood of respiratory problems prior to delivery?
b) What levels of blood sugar would you consider satisfactory?
c) What is the risk of the infant developing diabetes mellitus later on in life?

Answer to Question 78

a) Surfactant is relatively deficient in phosphatidyl glycerol (PG) and respiratory distress syndrome (RDS) may develop even in the presence of a normal lecithin/sphingomyelin ratio. To assess the risk of RDS either measure amniotic fluid PG levels or 'surfactant profile'.

b) 2.6 mmol/l Abnormal cerebral physiology is detected when blood glucose levels are below 2.6 mmol/l. Distinction between asymptomatic and symptomatic hypoglycaemia sometimes is difficult, and correction of persistent low blood glucose levels is necessary in 'asymptomatic' infants.

c) The risk to the infant of developing diabetes mellitus depends on the maternal type of diabetes preconceptionally; if she was an insulin-dependent diabetic, 1:33, or if NIDD, 1:10.

- Meticulous control of the maternal diabetes, ideally preconceptionally, reduces the acute postnatal problems but has not been shown to reduce the risk of congenital malformations.

- The incidence of macrosomia has been decreased with good antenatal control (up to 80%).

- Although hyperinsulinism is the main cause of hypoglycaemia, the diminished epinephrine and glucagon responses that occur may be contributing factors.

- True laboratory glucose measurements are mandatory when in doubt, as the 'reagent strips with the reflectance meter' method approximates by +/− 0.5 mmol/l the lab values.

- Rebound hypoglycaemia due to large boluses of hypertonic dextrose is common. It is due to the abnormal insulin response to a glucose load, seen in these infants. It should be avoided by using continuous infusions rather than boluses, when intravenous treatment is necessary to correct hypoglycaemia.

Aynsley–Green A 1992 Hypoglycaemia. In: David T J (ed) Recent advances in paediatrics, Vol 10, pp 37–62. Churchill Livingstone, Edinburgh
Becerra J E, Khoury M J, Cordero J F et al 1990 Diabetes mellitus during pregnancy and the risks for specific birth defects: a population based case control study. Paediatrics 85:1–9

Question 79

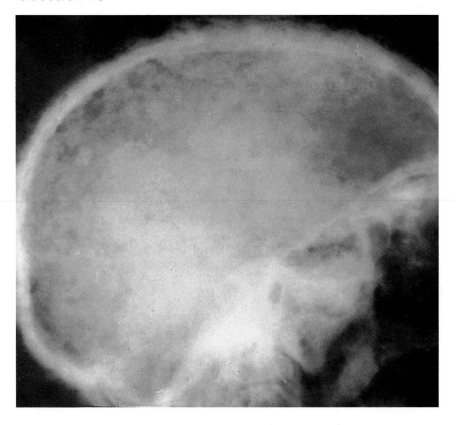

a) What is the diagnosis?
b) How do you confirm the diagnosis?
c) What is the appropriate counselling?

Answer to Question 79

a) B–thalassaemia major (the 'hairbrush' skull appearance caused by vertical trabeculae hypertrophy of erythropoietic tissue).

b) Hb electrophoresis; high levels of HbF >90%, no HbA and HbA–2 increased (or normal).

c) Cascade counselling: following the diagnosis of a case of B–thalassaemia major, identification of the heterozygote members of the family is essential for further genetic counselling.

- Current transfusion regimens are designed to minimize iron loading by maintaining an Hb level closer to normal (>10 g/dl).
- Haemosiderosis is delayed with adequate iron chelating therapy using desferrioxamine.
- Splenectomy performed as late as possible, when signs of hypersplenism appear, i.e. transfusion requirements exceed 240 ml/kg of packed cells/year.
- Serum ferritin is a good indicator of total body iron; levels <1000 ng/ml are considered non-toxic.
- For a select group of patients, who have a healthy HLA compatible sibling, allogenic bone marrow transplantation is an option.

Ehlers K H, Giardina P J et al 1991 Prolonged survival in patients with beta-thalassaemia major treated with desferrioxamine. J. Paediatr. 118:540–549

Question 80

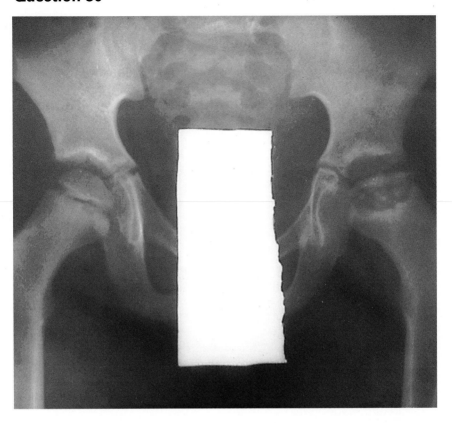

This is a radiograph of a 6-year-old boy with a recent history of a painful left hip and limp.

a) What is the diagnosis?
b) What is the differential diagnosis?
c) What is the treatment?

Answer to Question 80

a) Perthes disease.

b) Infection and trauma may jeopardize the blood supply to the capital epiphysis and cause varying degrees of ischaemic change; the history would usually exclude these differential diagnoses.

Infiltrative disease such as lymphoma deposits, Gaucher disease and eosinophilic granulomata may lead to obliterative vascular changes and necrosis of the femoral head.

c) The necrotic bone is gradually replaced by new bone, but recovery can be complicated by residual deformity of the femoral head. Containment in the acetabulum either by femoral osteotomy or bracing is occasionally required. The healing phase during which the head requires protection lasts 2 to 4 years.

- Perthes disease is a juvenile idiopathic avascular necrosis of the femoral head.
- Males are affected more than females (4–5:1).
- 20% of cases are familial.
- 10% of cases are bilateral.
- Early in the disease the bone scan is more sensitive than radiograms, showing decreased uptake; even more sensitive is magnetic resonance imaging (MRI), which demonstrates necrosis.
- The prognosis is usually good; half of the severe cases will require some joint replacement procedure at late middle adult life.
- Unfavourable factors are older age, complete involvement of the head and inadequate treatment.

Jani L, Hefti F 1990 Femur head necrosis in childhood. Orthopaede 19(4):191–199

Question 81

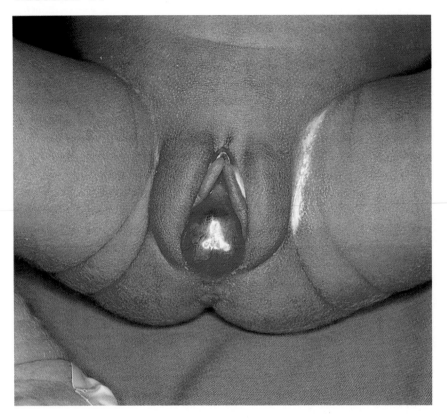

a) What is the differential diagnosis?
b) What investigation would you undertake?

Answer to Question 81

a) Ectopic ureter with a blind terminus
   Vaginal cyst
   Imperforate hymen with or without congenital hydrometrocolpos
   (distension of the uterus by retained secretions).
b) Abdominal ultrasound scan to check normality of the urinary tract,
   before incision and drainage of the cyst is performed.

Question 82

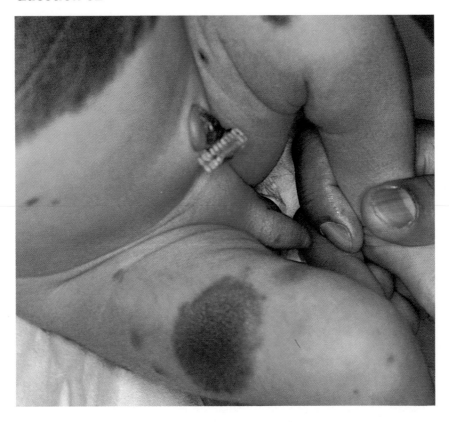

a) What is the diagnosis?
b) What particular risk is associated with this condition?
c) What is the recommended treatment?

Answer to Question 82

a) Giant congenital pigmented naevi (>20 cm).
b) The risk of malignant melanomatous transformation.
c) Total excision and grafting is the treatment of choice for giant naevi before 3 months of age. Dermabrasion is an alternative treatment.

- Giant (>20 cm) congenital pigmented naevi are very rare; 1:500 000 births.
- Melanocytic naevi, which are common later in childhood, are viewed with more concern when congenital, because they pose an increased risk over a lifetime for development of malignant melanoma. This risk applies for the large naevi of 20 cm or more and is estimated approximately at 10%.
- The lesions may be flat, elevated, verrucous or nodular, various shades of brown, blue or black and may develop numerous coarse hairs or may remain hairless and leathery.
- The histology is usually of an ordinary junctional, compound or intradermal naevus, and may differ in biopsy specimens obtained from several sites.
- In the neonate, all pigmented macules are not congenital naevi; the differential diagnosis includes mongolian spots, cafe-au-lait spots, smooth muscle hamartoma and dermal melanocytosis.
- There is considerable controversy concerning the appropriate approach to medium-sized (1.5–20 cm) congenital naevi. Rough estimates put the risk for melanomas between 0.8–4.9% until 60 years of age. It is now the prevailing opinion that they should be excised before adolescence.
- Early referral to paediatric dermatologists and plastic surgeons is advisable.

Ruiz–Maldonado R, Tamayo L et al 1992 Giant pigmented naevi: clinical, histopathologic and therapeutic considerations. J. Paediatr. 120:906–911

Question 83

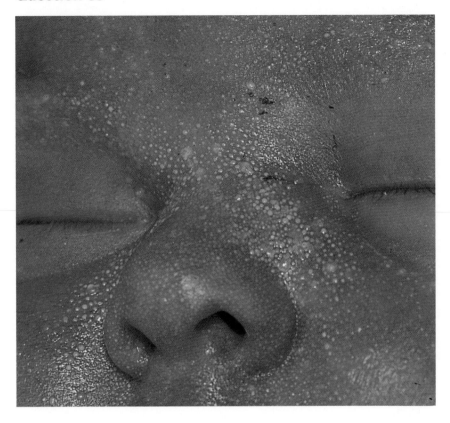

a) What is the diagnosis?
b) What is the natural history?

Answer to Question 83

a) Milia.
b) Although they may be very conspicuous in the first days of life, they disappear spontaneously after 3 to 4 weeks.

- These minute sebaceous cysts, which give rise to yellowish-white specks over the nose and face, are very common, found in about 40% of infants.
- Milia may occur at any age but in the neonate are most frequently scattered over the face and on the midline of the palate, when they are called Epstein pearls.
- Milia exfoliate spontaneously in most infants and may be ignored.

Question 84

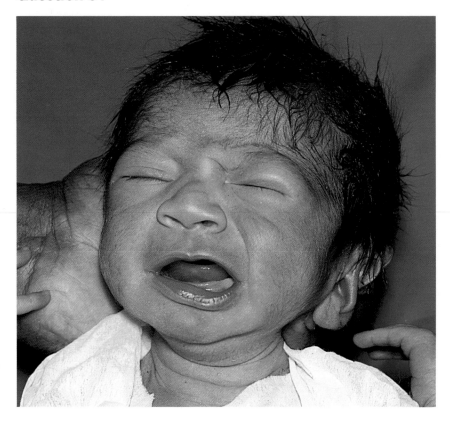

a) What is the diagnosis?
b) What is the treatment?
c) What is the prognosis?

Answer to Question 84

a) Right facial nerve palsy.
b) Usually no treatment is required, except perhaps the use of artifical tears for the open eye.
Rarely, feeding difficulties might require tube feeding.
c) When the facial palsy is a peripheral paralysis, resulting from pressure over the nerve during labour or instrumental delivery, then recovery is usually complete within days or weeks.

- Differential diagnosis includes intra-uterine pressure and congenital defects of the seventh nerve (e.g. nuclear agenesis), which is often bilateral, or other cranial nerves are affected; the prognosis for recovery of function in these cases is poor.
- Neuroplasty may be indicated when the paralysis is persistent.
- Facial palsy may be confused with the absence of the depressor muscles of the mouth, which is a benign condition.

Question 85

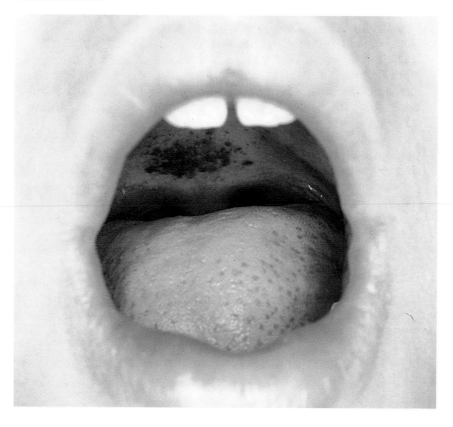

This 8-year-old boy presented to his family doctor with pyrexia, facial oedema, cervical lymphadenopathy and a mild splenomegaly.

a) What is the diagnosis?
b) How do you confirm the diagnosis?
c) What are the complications?

Answer to Question 85

a) Infectious mononucleosis (glandular fever).
b) Positive Paul–Bunnell test for heterophil antibodies
Epstein–Barr virus (EBV) specific serological studies.
c) Auto-immune haemolytic anaemia, thrombocytopenia, neurological complications (i.e. cranial nerve palsies, encephalitis), hepatitis, pericarditis, myocarditis, airway obstruction and splenic rupture.

- Heterophil antibodies are demonstrated in only 60% of children with glandular fever.
- Certain patients with EBV-induced mononucleosis, particularly pre-adolescents, or those with neurological complications may be heterophil-negative or may lack an atypical lymphocytosis.
- Neurological complications may be the presenting or sole manifestation of the disease.
- Airway obstruction from pharyngeal or paratracheal lymphadenopathy presents with acute stridor and is sensitive to steroids.
- The development of a maculopapular rash following the administration of ampicillin in patients with glandular fever is extremely common (80%); this rash is distinct from that associated with hypersensitivity to penicillins.

Chetham M M, Roberts K B 1991 Infectious mononucleosis in adolescents. Pediatr. Ann. 20(4):206–213

Question 86

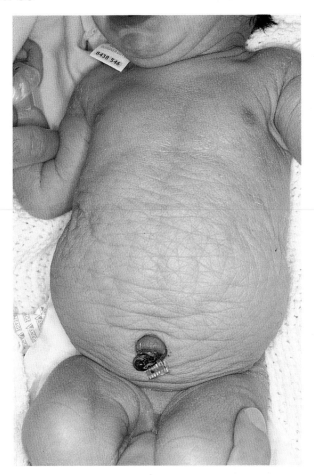

This female newborn presented with a transient tachypnoea soon after birth and remained anuric at 36 hours of age.

a) What is the likely diagnosis?
b) What urgent investigations would you undertake?
c) What is the differential diagnosis?

Answer to Question 86

a) Prune belly syndrome: the characteristic association of abdominal muscle deficiency, urinary tract abnormalities and undescended testes in the male.

b) Investigation of the urinary tract with a view to an urgent drainage procedure, if obstruction is complete.

c) As the newborn appears pink with a distended, baggy abdomen other conditions like congenital infections, fetal malignancies or liver disease should be excluded.

- Prune belly syndrome is rare, approximately 1:40 000.
- Oligohydramnios and pulmonary hypoplasia are frequent complications in the perinatal period.
- Many affected infants are stillborn.
- Only 3% of patients are females.
- Cardiac abnormalities occur in 10% of cases and more than 50% have abnormalities of the myoskeletal system.
- Urinary tract abnormalities are the most common cause of morbidity and medium/long term mortality; early mortality is usually due to pulmonary complications.
- Of the long term survivors, 50% develop chronic renal failure from dysplasia or reflux nephropathy; the results of renal transplantation in these patients are favourable.
- Correction of the undescended testes by orchidopexy is often difficult and is best accomplished in the first year of life.

Question 87

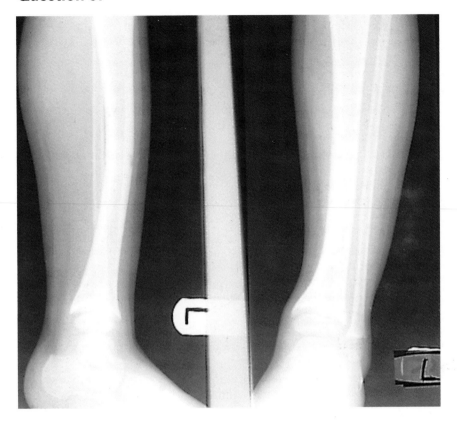

a) What is the diagnosis?
b) How would you confirm the diagnosis?
c) What is the aetiology of this condition?

Answer to Question 87

a) Rickets (deficient metaphyseal mineralization with irregular cupped bone margins).

b) Ca: normal or low
   P: low
   Alkaline phosphatase: high
   Vitamin D low
   25(OH) D low
   1.25(OH) D low.

c) The classic rickets is due to vitamin D deficiency, associated with lack of sunshine, skin pigmentation or poor diet.
   Secondary rickets may occur:
   Chronic liver disease, when 25 hydroxylation of vitamin D is impaired.
   Uncommonly in chronic renal failure, when the 1 hydroxylation of 25(OH) D to 1.25(OH) D is defective.
   Rarely during recovery from malabsorption.
   Prolonged therapy with anticonvulsants (mainly phenytoin), by induction of hepatic enzymes which degrade vitamin D to less active metabolites.
   Vitamin D resistant rickets (familial hypophosphataemic rickets, X-linked dominant condition), a defect in renal tubular transport of phosphate.
   Rickets complicating more general disorders of tubular function, i.e. RTA, Fanconi syndrome and cystinosis.

- The main antirachitic action of vitamin D is facilitation of intestinal absorption of calcium and phosphorus and of re-absorption of phosphorus in the kidney and a direct effect on mineral metabolism of bone (deposition and re-absorption).
- Rickets or epiphyseal dysplasia is particularly likely to develop during rapid growth, such as in low birth weight infants and in adolescents.

Reichel H, Koeffler H P et al 1989 The role of the vitamin D endocrine system in health and disease. N. Engl. J. Med. 320:980–991

Question 88

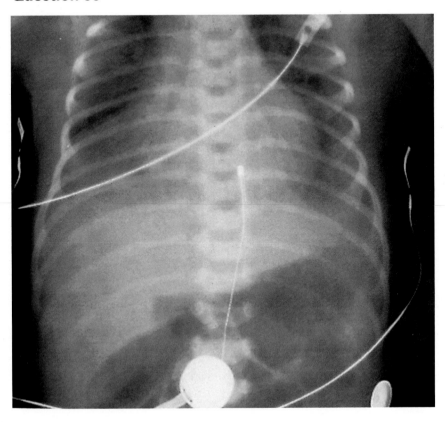

This is a 2-day-old neonate, born at 34 weeks' gestation, who required intubation and mechanical ventilation soon after birth for apnoea and cyanosis. There was meconium-stained liquor noted at delivery.

a) What is the diagnosis?
b) Give two likely pathogens in view of the history.
c) What additional pathology is evident on this chest radiograph?

Answer to Question 88

a) Right lower lobe congenital pneumonia.
b) Group B streptococcus (remains the commonest neonatal pathogen) *Listeria monocytogenes* (the history of meconium stained liquor in a preterm delivery suggests this causative organism).
c) Cardiomegaly without signs of fluid overload. Cardiac dysfunction with impaired ventricular function is not uncommon in septicaemia; often inotropic support with adequate preload is required.

- Congenital pneumonia is an important cause of morbidity and mortality; it is the most common inflammatory lesion found at autopsy in the neonatal period.
- Common bacterial pathogens are: Group B streptococcus, *E. coli, Listeria monocytogenes,* enterococci, klebsiella, *Haemophilus influenzae, Streptococcus pneumoniae,* etc.
- *Listeria monocytogenes* is best treated with ampicillin.
- Severe congenital pneumonia often becomes manifest as shock and profound hypoxia that is unresponsive to conventional ventilation and antibiotics. Extracorporeal membrane oxygenation may reverse the refractory hypoxia and improve cardiac output and oxygen delivery and has increased survival rates in the severest forms of congenital pneumonia to more than 70%.

Question 89

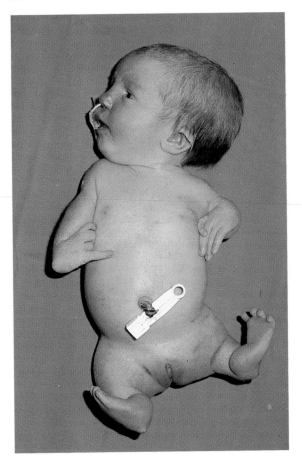

a) What is the diagnosis?
b) What is the type of inheritance?
c) What is the life expectancy?

Answer to Question 89

a) Thanatophoric dwarfism (Greek thanatos = death, phoros = bearing).

b) Affected siblings have been reported with normal parents, making autosomal recessive inheritance likely.

c) They usually die in the neonatal period from respiratory failure due to hypotonia and chest deformity.

- Thanatophoric dwarfism is a congenital chondrodystrophy of unknown aetiology, which is characterized by markedly shortened extremities, a relatively large head with associated hydrocephalus and a narrow thorax.
- It is the most frequent lethal congenital skeletal dysplasia.
- Infants with thanatophoric dwarfism are shorter at birth than those with achondroplasia.
- The changes in lumbar vertebrae are characteristic: inverted U shaped appearance in the AP view and marked flattening of the vertebrae with central narrowing in the lateral view.

Question 90

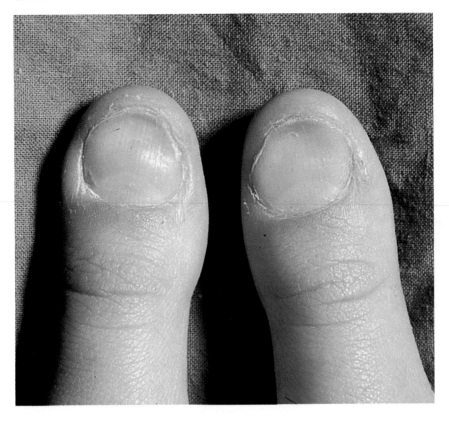

a) What is the physical sign demonstrated? Diagnosis?
b) What is the usual cause in early childhood?
c) How may the diagnosis be confirmed?

Answer to Question 90

a) Koilonychia due to iron deficiency anaemia.
b) Dietary factors.
c) By demonstrating a low Hb, hypochromic microcytosis and a low serum ferritin.

- The non-haematologic manifestations of iron deficiency, such as koilonychia, angular stomatitis and glossitis, are rarely seen nowadays, because iron deficiency anaemia (IDA) is more readily recognized and more promptly treated.
- In $1/3$ of cases of IDA occult blood is found in the stools.
- Thrombocytosis, sometimes of a striking degree, is not uncommon.
- Absent iron stores in the bone marrow aspirate make a definite diagnosis, but this is seldom required for diagnosis.
- The usual response to oral iron supplementation on IDA patients is: after 2–3 days reticulocytosis peaking at 5–7 days, elevation of the Hb from 4–30 days and repletion of iron stores in 1–3 months.
- If the response to iron supplementation is poor, compliance must be checked or other pathologies excluded by Hb electrophoresis, e.g. thalassaemia trait.
- Blood transfusion for severe IDA is usually unnecessary and may be dangerous; in the presence of heart failure not more than 2–3 ml/kg of packed cells should be given at a time. An exchange transfusion with packed cells can be an alternative.

Question 91

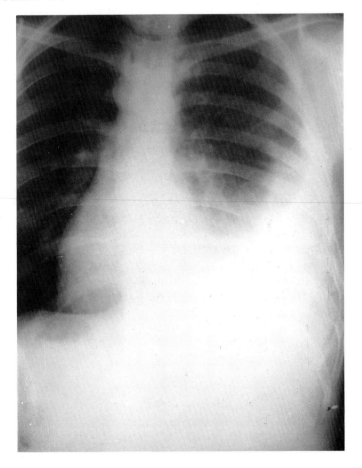

This 12-year-old boy presented with a 48 hour history of high fever and respiratory distress.

a) What is the likely diagnosis?
b) What is the prognosis?

Answer to Question 91

a) Pleural effusion secondary to pneumonia.
b) Prognosis for spontaneous resolution is very good.

- The most common cause of pleural effusion in children is bacterial pneumonia. Heart failure and metastatic intrathoracic malignancy are also well recognized aetiologies.
- *Staphylococcus aureus, Streptococcus penumoniae* and, in those under 5 years, *Haemophilus influenzae* are the most common bacteria associated with pleural effusion.
- Tuberculosis, although uncommon in the UK, should be considered and excluded.
- A secondary rise in the temperature in the course of a bacterial pneumonia is characteristic of the development of a pleural effusion, which may develop into an empyema.
- The fluid may be exudate, transudate, blood and chyle, depending on the primary pathology.
- Pleural effusions may be missed on supine films, when they produce a generalized hazy shadow on one or both lungs.

Question 92

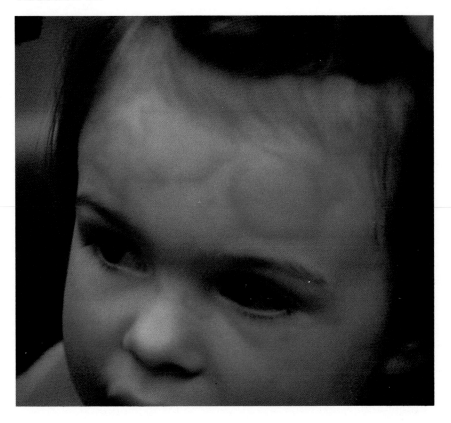

This toddler presented to her family doctor with a sore throat and swollen knees.

a) What is this lesion?
b) Give four common causes.
c) What is the treatment?

Answer to Question 92

a) Erythema multiforme.

b) Infections: *Herpes simplex,* coxsackie, haemolytic streptococcus, *Mycoplasma pneumoniae,* etc.
Drugs: penicillins, sulphonamides, barbiturates, aspirin, etc.
Miscellaneous causes: collagen disease, malignancies, vaccinations, radiotherapy.

c) Treatment tends to be symptomatic; steroids may be used when there is severe constitutional disturbance.

- Erythema multiforme (EM) is an acute, sometimes recurrent, inflammatory disease of the skin and mucous membranes. It is regarded as a hypersensitivity reaction triggered by drugs, infections and exposure to toxic substances.
- The cutaneous lesions are usually symmetrical, appear in crops and show a predilection for the palms and soles, extensor surfaces of the forearms and legs. As the disorder progresses, lesions often extend to the trunk, face and neck.
- Oral lesions may occur alone or in conjuction with cutaneous lesions.
- Despite the diversity of the mucocutaneous changes seen, usually there are annular red lesions with a purple centre, which in time show colour changes to resemble a bruise. When severe, these lesions show vesicular or even bullous formation.
- Severe constitutional disturbance with mucous membrane involvement and pyrexia is called Stevens–Johnson syndrome.
- Infection and occular lesions are the major cause of long term morbidity.
- Skin lesions usually heal with hypo- or hyperpigmentation after 4–6 weeks without scarring.
- Stevens–Johnson syndrome often requires intensive care treatment; superimposed bacterial infection is the leading cause of death.

Question 93

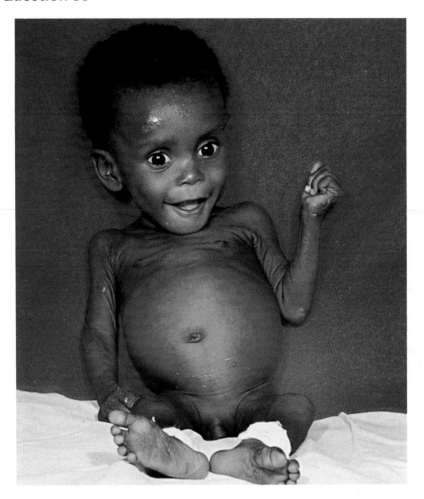

a) What is the likely diagnosis?
b) How do you diagnose early malnutrition in children?
c) What is the leading cause of death in this condition?

Answer 93

a) Marasmus (differs from kwashiorkor, as there is no oedema, dermatitis or sparse hair).

b) Severe disturbances are readily apparent, but mild ones may be overlooked. The diagnosis of malnutrition rests on:

Accurate dietary history

Evaluation of present deviations from average height, weight, head circumference and rates of growth

Circumference and rates of growth

Comparative measurements of midarm circumference and skinfold thickness

Chemical and other tests.

c) 'Common' infections, due to acquired immunodeficiency.

- Marasmus is severe malnutrition due to inadequate caloric intake, as opposed to kwashiorkor, which is protein malnutrition.
- Worldwide, malnutrition is one of the leading causes of morbidity and mortality in childhood.
- The clinical picture of marasmus is usually due to insufficient diet but can also be due to upset feeding habits, or to metabolic abnormalities or congenital malformations; severe impairment of any body system may result in malnutrition.
- Fat is lost last from the sucking pads of the cheeks, hence the infant's face may retain a relatively normal appearance for some time.
- The temperature is usually subnormal, the pulse may be slow and the basal metabolic rate tends to be reduced.
- After treatment has been initiated, the patient may lose weight for a few weeks, owing to loss of oedema.
- If growth and development have been extensively impaired, mental and physical retardation may be permanent; the younger the infant at the time of deprivation, the more devastating are the long term effects.
- Deficits in perceptual and abstract abilities are especially long-lasting.

Question 94

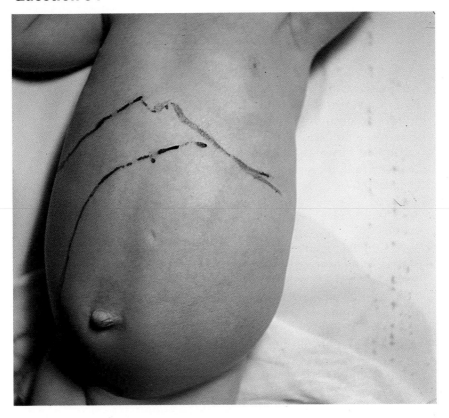

This infant presented with an abdominal mass and haematuria.

a) What is the likely diagnosis?
b) List three known associations.
c) What is the prognosis?

Answer to Question 94

a) Wilms tumour (nephroblastoma).

b) Urinary tract abnormalities–6%
Hemihypertophy–2–3%
Aniridia–1–2%
Also Beckwith syndrome, Bloom syndrome, von Hippel–Lindau syndrome, cerebral gigantism, bilateral retinoblastoma, neurofibromatosis, multiple pregnancy and undescended testes.

c) Survival is approximately 90% with localized resectable tumours; treatment includes chemotherapy followed by surgery and occasionally radiotherapy; if a child is disease-free after 2 years relapse is unlikely.

- Max Wilms was a German surgeon, who described the tumour in 1899.
- 5–10% of Wilms tumours are bilateral.
- Deletion of chromosome 11 has been noted in families of children with the aniridia–Wilms syndrome. It is consistently present at a submicroscopic level in cells of most Wilms tumours, even when the constitutional chromosomal composition is normal.
- The familial form is more likely to be bilateral than the sporadic form.
- The risk of Wilms tumour in the offsprings of a patient with bilateral or familial Wilms tumour is approximately 30%.
- Hypertension is detected in up to 60% of patients due to renal ischaemia, resulting from the pressure of the tumour on the renal artery; it may result in congestive heart failure.
- The major differential diagnosis is neuroblastoma; CT will establish the intrarenal origin of the tumour.
- Pulmonary metastases are present in 10–15% at time of diagnosis.
- Pre-operative therapy is not recommended for patients with unilateral disease.
- Prognosis is better when diagnosis occurs before the age of 2 years and tumour weight is less than 250g. The most significant prognostic variables are histology and stage.
- Bloom syndrome comprises facial telangiectasia with a butterfly distribution, short stature and photosensitivity. Von Hippel–Lindau syndrome comprises retinal changes with cerebellar ataxia.

Question 95

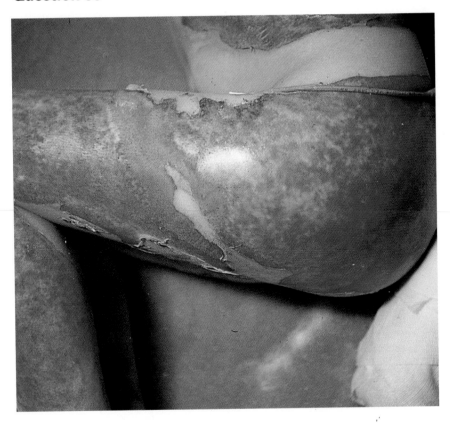

a) Describe your immediate management of this patient.
b) Give three common complications.

Answer to Question 95

a) Maintain patent airway and adequate ventilation
Maintain adequate intravascular volume; colloids are commonly
needed (avoid overhydration)
Sedation and adequate analgesia
Empty the stomach; consider stress ulcers
Antitetanus prophylaxis and antibiotic cover

b) Cardiac dysfunction: the myocardial depressant factor (MDF),
a circulating substance identified in severely burned patients,
decreases contractility and reduces cardiac output. Congestive
heart failure and pulmonary oedema may ensue
Respiratory problems are common, particularly with smoke inhala-
tion or facial burns
Renal failure (usually of prerenal aetiology)
Sepsis: increased susceptibility due to the loss of the skin barrier,
plus defects in host resistance.

- Burns are the leading cause of accidental death at home among
  children aged 1–4 years.
- Substantial burns exceeding 10% of body surface and burns involv-
  ing the face, hands, feet or genitalia are indications for hospital
  admission.
- Non-accidental injury should be suspected when the history and
  the physical findings are inconsistent, bizarre or recurrent.

Question 96

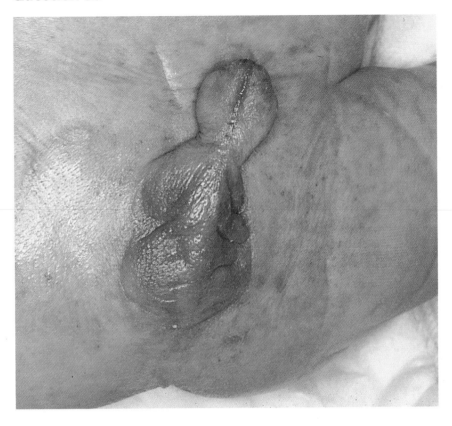

a) What abnormalities are shown?
b) What are the two priorities in this condition?
c) What urgent investigations would you undertake?

Answer to Question 96

a) Ambiguous genitalia with bilateral cryptorchidism
b) To establish the appropriate gender
  To recognize life-threatening complications, notably salt-losing congenital adrenal hyperplasia (CAH)
c) Urgent pelvic ultrasound or radiology to assess pelvic organs and gonads
  Chromosomal karyotype and investigations to exclude CAH
  Look for palpable gonads. Gonads in the lower inguinal or scrotal region are virtually always testicular and this finding rules out simple virilization of females.

- The incidence of cryptorchidism is approximately 3% in full term babies and 30% in premature ones.
- Spontaneous descent of the testes is possible during the first year of life, leaving approximately 1:100 requiring surgery.
- Infertility in adulthood, tumour development in the undescended testes, associated hernias, testicular torsion and psychological effects are all potential consequences of cryptorchidism.
- The undescended testis is often histologically normal at birth, but failure of development and atrophy are detectable by the end of the first year of life and after the second year the number of germ cells in the affected testis is severely reduced.
- Early surgery is the current approach.

Question 97

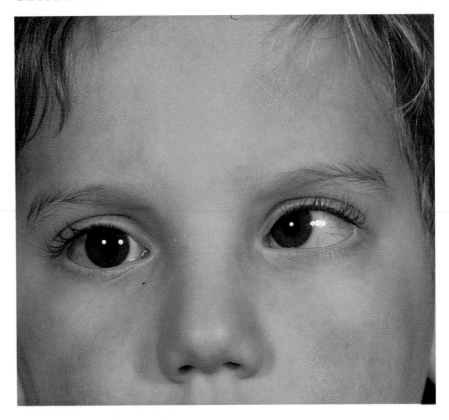

a) What is the diagnosis?
b) Which cases do you select for ophthalmic referral?
c) What are the common associations of this condition?

Answer to Question 97

a) Left convergent squint.

b) Squints are common in the neonatal period; all need basic ophthalmoscopy, including the red reflex. Prompt ophthalmic referral for all fixed or divergent squints or infantile squints persisting longer than 4–6 months from birth.

c) Refractive errors, particularly hypermetropia and astigmatism
Neurological disorders interfering with the normal function of the extra-ocular muscles
Eye diseases like cataracts or retinoblastoma.

- Pseudo-squint is common, usually due to marked epicanthal folds, a broad nasal bridge or other facial asymmetries. They improve in time as these asymmetries lessen with growth.
- The goal of treatment for squint is to develop the best possible vision with optimal ocular alignment, especially for the forward gaze position.
- Underlying defects such as cataracts must be corrected with lenses and any amblyopia must be vigorously treated with occlusion of the 'good' eye.

Elkington A R, Khaw P T 1988 Squint. Br. Med. J. 297:608–611
Fielder A R 1989 The management of squint. Arch. Dis. Child. 64:413–418

Question 98

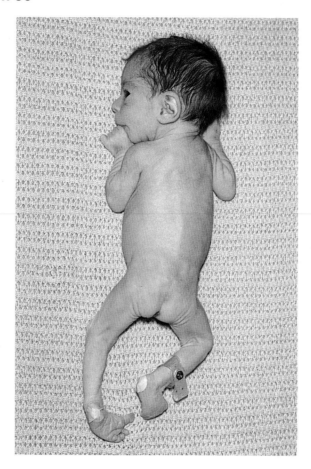

a) What is the diagnosis?
b) Give three common perinatal problems in this particular condition.
c) What is the appropriate postnatal management?

Answer to Question 98

a) Asymmetrical intra-uterine growth retardation (IUGR)

b) Birth asphyxia: Mild intrapartum asphyxia may cause severe effects, because of the poor fat and glycogen stores and thus poor ability to maintain anaerobic metabolism

Hypoglycaemia: reasons as above; it usually peaks at 24–48 hours postnatally, particularly if the infant is breastfed (hypocaloric intake), when the body stores of fat and glycogen have been consumed. Severe IUGR babies can develop neuroglycopenia much earlier

Hypocalcaemia

Hypothermia: due to large surface area to body volume

Polycythaemia, thrombocytopenia

Meconium aspiration

Pulmonary haemorrhage

Necrotizing enterocolitis

c) Prevent any cold stress

If the newborn is asymptomatic start early and frequent feeds under BMStix monitoring; if symptomatic, use adequate dextrose i.v. infusions

- There are two groups of small-for-dates infants: the proportionately growth retarded infant for gestation, suggesting early onset of IUGR, and the asymmetrical IUGR infant, suggesting recent onset of IUGR.
- Common causes of asymmetrical IUGR are placental insufficiency, pre-eclampsia, maternal smoking, etc.
- The prognosis for IUGR infants depends on the aetiology of their growth retardation and on the acute management of potential neonatal problems.

Question 99

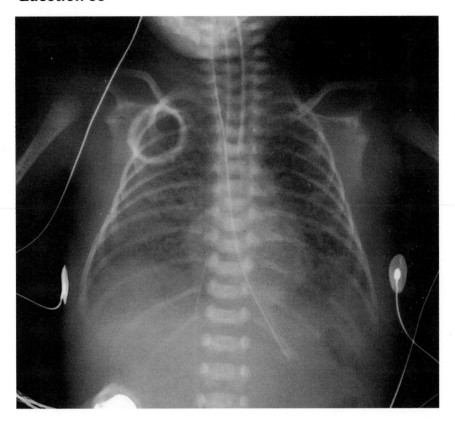

This premature baby required ventilation soon after birth for progressive respiratory distress. His lecithin to sphingomyelin ratio (L/S) on gastric aspirate was 0.9.

a) What is the most likely diagnosis?
b) What antenatal management prior to preterm delivery may help to ameliorate this infant's diagnosis?

Answer to Question 99

a) Hyaline membrane disease (HMD).

b) Antenatal glucocorticoid therapy (dexamethasone) accelerates surfactant production in preterm infants, particularly at 30–34 weeks'
gestation. Additional benefit may be gained from the concurrent
administration of thyrotropin releasing hormone (TRH).

- Surfactant and Type II pneumocytes appear in the human lung at
  about 20 weeks' gestation. Initially a slow increase is observed, until
  the 30–34 weeks' gestation, when a significant surge occurs.
- Surfactant production postnatally is reduced in the presence of
  hypothermia, hypoxia and acidosis.
- Intra-uterine stress, premature rupture of the membranes or maternal hypertension can stimulate surfactant production, possibly due
  to the release of endogenous steroid from the fetal adrenal glands.
- The lungs may have a characteristic but no pathognomonic radiological appearance; the severity of the radiological changes often
  reflects the severity of the HMD.
- Exogenous surfactant administration is an adjunct to conventional
  management of HMD with proven efficacy on very preterm babies
  and, in some studies, in larger babies weighing >1250g.

Yu V Y H 1986 Respiratory distress syndrome. In: Yu V Y H (ed)
Respiratory disorders in the newborn. Churchill Livingstone,
Edinburgh

Question 100

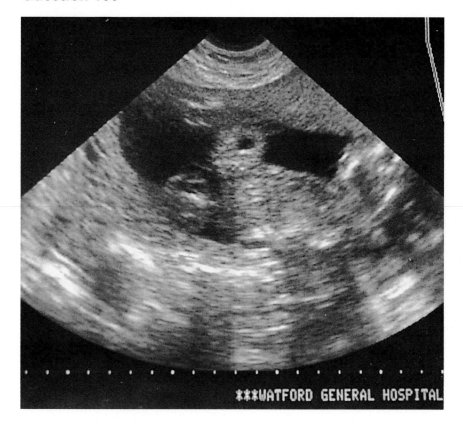

This is an antenatal ultrasound at 24 weeks' gestation.

a) What abnormality is shown?
b) What is a frequent association with this defect?
c) What is the recommended mode of delivery?

Answer to Question 100

a) Exomphalos (omphalocele).
b) Beckwith–Wiedemann syndrome; the diagnosis is strongly suspected antenatally when ultrasonography demonstrates exomphalos, associated with macrosomia, organomegaly and macroglossia.
c) Elective caesarean section is not advantageous; vaginal delivery with optimal neonatal care appears as safe.

- Exomphalos is the herniation or protrusion of abdominal contents into the base of the umbilical cord.
- The incidence varies from 1:5000 births (intestines into the cord) to 1:10 000 (liver and intestines).
- It develops between 8 and 10 weeks and is due to failure of the eventrated gut to return into the abdominal cavity during its development.
- Exomphalos is shown by the presence of a mass, cystic if it contains loops of bowel, or echodense if it contains liver; It is situated on the anterior abdominal wall and bears a constant relationship to the fetal trunk.

Lewis D F, Towers C V et al 1990 Fetal gastroschisis and omphalocele: is caesarean section the best mode of delivery? Amer. J. Obst. Gyn. 163(3):773–775
Roberts J P, Burge D M 1990 Antenatal diagnosis of abdominal wall defects: a missed opportunity? Arch. Dis. Child. 65:687–689

INDEX TO QUESTIONS

Abscess, pulmonary 31
Adrenal hyperplasia, congenital 5
Ambiguous genitalia 5, 96
Amniotic bands 61
Anaemia, iron deficiency 90
Angelman syndrome 9
Angio-oedema 35
Ascites 11

BCG 53
Beckwith–Wiedemann syndrome 71, 100
Bernard Soulier syndrome 51
Bites 41
Bronchopulmonary dysplasia 50
Burns 95

Cardiac disease, congenital 69
Cardiomegaly 27
Cellulitis 19
Cephalhaematoma 39, 68
Chromosomal abnormalities 9, 21, 23,
    24, 40, 47, 71
Cleft lip 56
Clinodactyly 46
Clubbing 46
Cranial nerve palsy 25, 84
Craniosynostosis 33
Cystic fibrosis 49, 52

Down syndrome 21, 24

Ears, low set 42
Ecchymoses 48
Ectodermal dysplasia 54
Ectrodactyly 54
Eczema herpeticum 16
Edwards syndrome 23, 40
EEC syndrome 54
Encephalocele 58
Erb palsy 30
Erythema marginatum 14
         multiforme 92
         nodosum 8
Exomphalos 63, 100

Facial nerve palsy 84
Foreign body 59

Gastroschisis 63, 70
Genitalia, ambiguous 5, 96
Group B streptococcal disease 64

Haemangioma 34
Hemorrhagic shock & encephalopathy
    syndrome 48
Henoch-Schönlein purpura 2
Hirschsprung disease 13
Hyaline membrane disease 64, 99
Hydro-ureter 62
Hypoglycaemia 78
Hypothyroidism, congenital 18
Hypotonia 37

Impetigo 44
Infectious mononucleosis 85
Intra-uterine growth retardation 98
Intussusception 2, 3

Juvenile chronic arthritis 45

Kawasaki syndrome 75
Koilonychia 90

Lung abscess 31
Lymphangioma 12

Marasmus 93
Meningitis 25
Meningococcal sepsis 4, 17
Meningomyelocele 22
Milia 83
Mongolian blue spot 32
Mycoplasma infection 76
Myopathy 37

Naevi giant hairy 26
      melanocytic 82
Necrotizing enterocolitis 13

Omphalocele 63, 100
Osteogenesis imperfecta 29
Osteomyelitis 6
Osteopetrosis 10

Patau syndrome 40

Pendred syndrome 18
Periventricular leucomalacia 1
Perthes disease 80
Pertussis 28, 73
Petechiae 28, 85
Photo-erythema 44
Phytophotodermatitis 38
Pleural effusion 91
Pneumonitis 65
Pneumonia 15, 76, 88
Pneumothorax 20
Potter syndrome 42
Prune belly syndrome 86
Pseudo Bartter syndrome 52
Pulmonary abscess 31
Purpura fulminans 4
            Henoch–Schönlein 2
            thrombocytopenic 43,
            74
Pyknodysostosis 57
Pyloric stenosis 60

Rickets 87
Rockerbottom feet 23, 40

Scaphocephaly 33
Sclerosing peritonitis 11
Sickle cell disease 15, 27
Skeletal dysplasia 55
Squint 97
Staphylococcal disease 19, 44
Strabismus 97

Thalassaemia major 79
Thanatophoric dwarfism 89
Thrombocytopenic purpura 43, 74
Thyroglossal cyst 36
Tooth, congenital 66
Toxic shock syndrome 44
Toxoplasmosis, congenital 77
Transfusion, twin–twin 7
Tuberous sclerosis 67
Turner syndrome 42

Urticaria 35

Vaginal cyst 81
Ventriculoseptal defect 72

Wilms tumour 94